The Vagus N
Body's Su

Simple Three-Minute Exercises to
Activate Your Body's Natural Healing
Power to Relieve Inflammation,
Stress, Anxiety, Depression, and
Chronic Illness

Galen Hart

Table of Contents

Introduction

There is no denying anxiety, depression, and chronic stress are taking over far too many lives: In the United States alone, more than 40 million adults struggle with anxiety (National Alliance on Mental Illness, 2017). Shockingly, 2020 saw 21 million adults suffer from at least one depressive episode during the year (National Alliance on Mental Health, 2022). Unfortunately, these mental imbalances are not exclusive to adults: Children, too, are suffering from anxiety disorders, depression, and chronic illness. The unrelenting pressure of our daily lives is taking its toll on the lives of countless people, and the statistics are there to prove it.

These mental imbalances have serious consequences, not just for individuals, but for our society at large. In a human being, stress can cause illness and reduced productivity, which in turn has an effect on personal and professional relationships, as well as financial security and future certainty. Physical symptoms of mental imbalances include changes in appetite, reduced metabolism, headaches, digestive problems, muscle tension, decreased immunity, difficulty sleeping, and a whole host of other health-related problems. Mental imbalances also influence our emotional responses and cognitive abilities. Being overwhelmed by our circumstances can lead to outbursts of anger, low levels of energy, difficulty with memory and focus, and a lack of motivation. A 2020 survey by the American Psychological Association revealed that Americans were facing a mental health crisis of national proportions that cost the government billions of dollars. People are unable to show up to work, workplace accidents are on the rise, children can no longer go to school, and the death toll keeps rising as a result of stress-related diseases… and the cause is that everyone suffers the consequences of mental imbalances, whether it's on a personal, professional, or even institutional level.

There is an increasing amount of information out there about how to remain healthy physically, mentally, and emotionally, so why does it seem as if mental imbalances are becoming more and more prevalent with each passing day? The most obvious guess is that our lives are simply too busy. People have to deal with work stress, financial problems, health issues, children, partners, friends, and coworkers—and it's simply too overwhelming for the majority of individuals. Another reason might be that we're always "plugged in:" We are in constant contact with the rest of the world 24 hours a day, and most of the time, it's impossible to get away from negativity and bad news. Political turmoil, economic upheaval, social disparities and oppression, climate change, harmful marketing tactics. It's no wonder people have such difficulty holding on to their health and happiness. Furthermore, although people seem to be more knowledgeable than ever about mental imbalances, we lack examples of people who are capable of healthy emotional processing and stress management. Few people are able to find balance in their lives, and they have no one to look up to when they become overwhelmed.

The consequence of the society we've bought into is that emotional dysregulation has become nearly commonplace. We've not been given healthy and effective ways to deal with our stress and manage our emotions, anxiety, and depression, which have made chronic illness mainstream. Ironically, while our circumstances lie at the root of our mental imbalances, having these imbalances increases our stress—and this makes life even more difficult. Living with anxiety, depression, and chronic illness looks different in every individual: Some people display physical symptoms such as illnesses and diseases, while others tend to isolate themselves, or have difficulty navigating social situations. Mental imbalances can also lead to substance abuse, eating disorders, and other mental illnesses that stem from being under constant pressure. Whatever your experience is, there is a way to self-regulate and relieve your symptoms.

The good news is that self-regulation is within your reach with the right tools and resources. My goal is to teach you holistic strategies to manage pain and ease your symptoms by testing and toning your vagus nerve, which is your body's superpower. By cultivating a sense of self-awareness and mindfulness, and harnessing the power of your vagus nerve, you can learn to reduce your anxiety, depression, and stress in the long-term.

I have been a teacher for 25 years: I have always been interested in nutrition, health, and naturopathy, and while I believe there is a time and place for medication, my personal belief is that it's always better to heal yourself naturally as much as possible. Unknowingly, I used bits and pieces of polyvagal theory for years while healing my own health issues, and I continue to be amazed at the human body's capacity to heal itself. We now know that your mind and body don't work as separate entities, but that they function as one complex ecosystem in which each part can affect another, and none of them can work by themselves.

Ten years ago, I suffered from bilateral carpal tunnel syndrome accompanied by nerve damage. Despite many attempts, Western medicine simply couldn't heal these ailments. For two years, I tried everything I could find; eventually, I turned to biofeedback, medical massage, and acupuncture. Biofeedback taught me to calm my nervous system through breathwork, and medical massage of my neck and shoulders helped to reduce my pain. What I didn't know at the time was that these practices have been shown to improve vagal tone. As for acupuncture, I was amazed at how quickly it addressed the pain and healed my injury. Although I didn't understand it, I was grateful for the relief. I have since learned that there are many studies that show that acupuncture can also help stimulate the vagus nerve, which in turn has anti-inflammatory effects on the body.

In addition to relieving my physical pain, toning my vagus nerve also helped me to deal with my mental imbalances. I went through a long and difficult divorce that caused a lot of anxiety and depression for me. The only place where I felt I could breathe deeply and be released from my anxiety during this time was in yoga class. Of course, I didn't realize the reason for this was because yoga was stimulating my vagus nerve. When I went through a battle with breast cancer, yoga rescued me once again. I felt alone and scared, and yoga class became a safe zone for me where I could truly relax. I didn't understand why this was my experience, but activating my vagus nerve was, in reality, relieving my stress. Nowadays, I do yoga and breathwork almost every day, because I continue to love the way it makes me feel.

I have a lot more knowledge now than I did in the past, but it has occurred to me that if I'd had this information earlier, I would have been able to recover faster—and this is why I'm so passionate about sharing what I know with others. Please keep in mind I am not a doctor and I can't offer professional medical advice. I can, however, share my own story of recovery, a lay person's perspective on holistic healing in general, and my own experience with vagal healing specifically. Remember to seek your doctor's advice about your health concerns before you start any new routine.

My goal is to put people in control of their bodies by teaching them how to use the vagus nerve to stop the typical cycle of *fight or flight*, and to bring them into the *rest and digest* mode. Only then, does the body feel relaxed and safe enough to start the healing process and attain optimal health. It has helped me turn my life around, and it continues to be the thing I turn to when something in my body is amiss. Not only has it proven extremely effective, but it's also so easy, it almost feels illegal!

Society continues to move forward, as it should, and many of us do not have the luxury of scaling down. However, we can learn ways to harness the vagus nerve to help us handle stress so that it does not severely impact our bodies. We are not alone: There are thousands of people like us who struggle every day to stay healthy and function more efficiently. Keep reading for more knowledge about the 10th cranial nerve, or if you are not curious about the science behind the vagus nerve feel free to skip straight to Chapter 7, where you will find simple exercises that you can do to tone your vagus nerve!

Chapter 1:

What Is the Vagus Nerve?

The first step to understanding how your vagus nerve can heal your body is, of course, to understand what the vagus nerve is. The purpose of this chapter is to outline a few basic ideas around nerves in general, and vagal nerves specifically. As an introduction to information about the vagus nerve, it discusses:

- What is neurology, and why it's important for us to understand.

- What nerves are and how they work.

- The difference between cranial nerves and spinal nerves.

- What the vagus nerve is.

- Where the vagus nerve is located.

- What the role of vagal nerves are in your body's overall functioning.

- What nerves look like, and how they communicate with each other.

It's important to remember that nerves and the nervous system—and the vagus nerves in particular—is a complex field of study. That being said, for the purposes of this journey, it's possible to try and keep things as simple as possible.

What, Where, and Why?

Human Neurology

Neurology is the study of the brain, spinal cord, and nerves as far as the nervous system is concerned. It is also concerned with treating disorders and diseases of the nervous system. Our nervous system is our body's communication system, and is responsible for nearly everything that happens to us on a physical, emotional, and mental level. Think of your nervous system as your "wiring:" Without it, nothing in your body— including your muscles, senses, and organs—would be able to function. Even worse, if your wiring is faulty, it can have serious consequences for your mental and physical health.

Neurology is a specialized medical field that is practiced by trained neurologists, and it takes many years of dedication and hard work to come to a full understanding of how the nervous system works, how dysregulation can be diagnosed, and what treatments are available for those who are suffering from nervous system disorders. That being said, it can't hurt for all of us to come to a better understanding of how our physiology functions. More importantly, given the inescapable role that our nervous systems play in our overall functioning, it's essential that we dig a little deeper into the mystery that is our bodies.

Nerves, and the Vagus Nerve

Take a look at your hand, imagine lifting it into the air. Now do it: Watch it rise away from you, feel your muscles tense as it lifts, take in the temperature as you move it through the air, feel the texture of your skin, your fingers, the palm of your hand… how did you do that? How did your muscles know what you were thinking, and how did your brain know what your hand was feeling? The answer: Nerves.

Nerves are fibers in your body that carry messages between your brain and the rest of your body. In other words, they are responsible for all the communication that happens between the different parts of your body, as well as your responses to anything that happens outside of yourself. If you touch something hot, for instance, the nerves in your fingers will transmit this message to your brain, which is translated into the burning you feel. In turn, signals between your brain and your hand will activate the muscles in your arm, making you move your hand away from the thing that's burning you. Similarly, if you think of doing something—speaking, walking, swallowing—your brain will communicate this to the right muscles, and this will transform your thoughts into external action. As a communication system, your nerves are the connection between the countless elements that your body is made up of, including your brain, spinal cord, organs, glands, muscles, and skin.

There are a number of different types of nerves, and each controls a distinct function in your body. Nerves, for example, are responsible for your senses, appetite and metabolism, balance and coordination, muscular activity, breathing, digestion, heart rate, involuntary reflexes, glandular activity, cognitive and emotional capabilities, immunity, aging, stress responses, and our ability to rest, relax, and sleep. Two of the main nerve types are *motor nerves*—which are what makes movement possible—and *sensory nerves,* which are the reason why you're able to use parts of your body to experience senses. In other words, your nerves are the reason you're able to do everything you do, every day.

Your nerves can be *efferent*, which means they're responsible for transmitting messages outward from your brain and spinal cord to your other organs. In contrast, they can also be *afferent,* which means they communicate information from your organs or your external environment to your brain and spinal cord. This means that the nervous system is a two-way communication system that both transmits and receives messages through the body. Furthermore, these messages can originate in your body, but they can also be triggered by your outward environment. The external or internal factor that triggers a nerve to send a message is known as a *stimulus*. A soundwave, for example, is a stimulus that stimulates nerves in your ears to send a message to your brain, which is then transformed into a sound you're able to make sense of. Similarly, unintelligible light waves trigger nerves in your eye to translate them into something your brain can recognize, and therefore see. It's important to remember that the responses created by your nerves are involuntary; in other words, you can't control how you will react to internal or external stimuli.

The two biggest role-players in your nervous system are your spinal cord and your brain, but nerves are located throughout your body, from your little toe all the way to the top of your head. To simplify their organization, they have been divided into two types: Cranial nerves and spinal nerves. Cranial nerves originate in the brain, and control many functions that occur throughout your body. For instance, your cranial nerves are responsible for your sense of taste and smell, as well as your vision, balance, hearing, facial expressions, tongue movements. They are also responsible for your cognition and perception, and are the reason you're able to think, remember, create, and reason. Spinal nerves, on the other hand, originate in the spinal cord, and they branch out to the rest of your body. These are the nerves that are responsible for the sensations you feel in your lower body, as well as any organ, glandular, and muscle movement in this region.

Neuroception is the process by which neural circuits determine whether a situation is life-threatening, or a person is safe or in danger. Unlike perception, which is a cognitive thought, neuroception involves brain processes that work beyond our conscious awareness.

Your body has 30 different spinal nerves and 12 types of cranial nerves, of which the vagus nerve—or cranial nerve X—is the longest. *Vagus* is the Latin word for "wanderer" in English; this is a good description of this nerve, as it stretches from your brain all the way to your abdomen. It's not without reason that the vagus nerve is described as the body's "superhighway" of communication: It is the connection between your brain and a multitude of organs, including your lungs, liver, gut, intestines, heart, spleen, and kidneys. It is also the backbone of the "gut-brain axis," which is described in more detail in Chapter 3.

The path of the wandering nerve starts in your brain. From there, it travels to your throat—or more specifically, your pharynx and larynx. Here, it is responsible for your ability to swallow, speak, cough, sneeze, and vomit. From your throat, it moves into your chest, where it controls your breathing and heart rate. As it wanders downward, it passes through your gut, where it impacts your digestion and elimination processes. It is also here in the gut where it influences your immune system. But how are these organs connected to your mood and emotional responses? Simply put, your vagus nerve is responsible for calming your body down, or reregulating your system after a scare or a shock. If these functions are dysregulated, you will remain in fight-or-flight mode chronically, and this could impact your mental health. The impact of your vagus nerve on your mood is discussed in more detail in Chapters 3 and 4.

It is the vagus nerve's extensive reach that makes it your body's superpower, and the key to healing mental imbalances and self-regulation. The tenth cranial nerve—the vagus nerve—begins at the base of your brain. It is a single nerve that branches out to form two parts that feather out and down, touching all of your internal organs. This means the vagus nerve is responsible for a vast array of messages from all over your body, both toward and away from your brain. In addition, it also means that there are several unlikely parts of your body—such as your gut and your brain—that are connected to each other in unexpected but significant ways.

How Do Nerves Communicate?

For many years, nobody knew how the various parts of the human body communicated with each other. However, in 1921, physiologist, Otto Loewi, had a dream—literally—about an experiment that later came to confirm nerve communication. Using frog hearts and a saline solution, Loewski slowed down the heart rate of one of the frogs by stimulating its vagus nerve. When he transferred this saline solution to the other heart, he found that its heart rate slowed down, too. This led him to conclude that a substance was released by the vagus nerve of the first heart, and that this chemical communicated a message to the second heart. In this fashion, it was discovered that nerves transmit messages by means of chemicals, known as *neurotransmitters*. Different nerves release different types of chemicals, but the vagus nerve in particular makes use of a substance known as *acetylcholine* to communicate with the rest of the body.

In addition to chemical messages, nerves also use electrical signals to communicate with each other. This is possible because of the very specific composition of nerves. There are endless types of nerves, all serving a different function. Even the most basic nerve is made up of cells known as *neurons*. Neurons can either be classified as motor or sensory—as mentioned above—or as interneurons, which are what connects a string of neurons to each other. Every neuron has a cell body that drives the entire neuron structure, and that can be thought of as the "powerhouse" of the cell. The nucleus— or center—of the cell body is connected to a number of thin fibers called *dendrites*. These are short, branching structures, and they are what transmits messages to the neuron from its adjacent neighbors. In addition, every neuron also has a single, long *axon* that sends messages away from the nucleus of the cell body. When an organ is triggered by a stimulus, it causes electrochemical pulses to travel from the cell body of one neuron to the cell body of its neighbor along the chain of axons and dendrites. There are variations on this composition depending on the function of the nerve, but generally speaking, this is how the body is able to transmit messages from one organ to another.

Like the rest of your body, your nerves and their individual elements are subject to damage and injury. Given their importance in your body's overall functioning, this can have serious consequences for your mental and physical health. The vagus nerve, in particular, can cause a whole host of problems if it becomes dysregulated; this is discussed in more detail in Chapter 2.

Chapter 2:

The Nervous System and the

Vagus Nerve

The vagus nerve is one of the largest and most important nerves in our bodies. That being said, it forms part of a much larger system—known as our nervous system—and to understand how the vagus nerve can influence your body, you first have to understand how it fits in with the rest of the nervous system. This chapter therefore discusses:

- The nervous system, its division into the central nervous system and peripheral nervous system, and what the purpose of each of these is.

- The division of the peripheral nervous system into the somatic nervous system and the autonomic nervous system (ANS), and how each of these functions.

- The role and mechanisms of the enteric, sympathetic, and parasympathetic nervous systems as different parts of the autonomic nervous system.

- What autonomic functioning means.

- The differences between a regulated and dysregulated body, and the physical and mental symptoms associated with each.

- How mental imbalances occur as a result of autonomic dysregulation.

- The role of the vagus nerve in mental imbalances—such as anxiety, depression, and chronic stress—and how this affects our emotional responses.

- The role of the vagus nerve in the gut-brain axis.

The Nervous System

The Sympathetic and Parasympathetic Nervous Systems

The ANS is responsible for a wide range of bodily functions, which are divided into, and controlled by, three parts: The enteric nervous system, the sympathetic nervous system, and the parasympathetic nervous system. The *enteric nervous system*—or ENT—is mostly related to digestion, and it controls saliva production, bodily secretions such as sweat, and blood flow. It is also responsible for activity in the endocrine system, which is a network of glands that release hormones into the body. It works mostly in isolation, but there is some interaction between the ENT and the sympathetic and parasympathetic nervous systems. In contrast, the sympathetic and parasympathetic nervous systems work together at all times—albeit in opposite directions.

The Sympathetic Nervous System

The *sympathetic nervous system* is what your body turns to when it finds itself in "fight-or-flight" situations where it requires increased activity, a sense of alertness, or a certain amount of strength. Your sympathetic nervous system is responsible for feelings such as fear, embarrassment, anger, or excitement, because it creates the physical responses we associate with these feelings. For instance, when you find yourself in danger, your breathing rate and heart rate will increase, and you may become sweaty and hot. This is because the nerves in your sympathetic nervous system are activating the muscles in your lungs and heart by dilating the blood vessels that supply blood to these organs, so that they receive more oxygen. They also trigger the sweat glands and the adrenal glands—which then release adrenaline into your system—and dilate the blood vessels of your skin so that you become flushed, or get goose bumps. They may allow more blood to flow to other muscles so that you become physically stronger, and release more glucose into your system to increase your energy levels. The sympathetic nervous system is also responsible for improving your eyesight in stressful situations by dilating your pupils to allow additional light into your eyes. In addition to increasing the body's activity level and preparing it for high-energy conditions, the sympathetic nervous system also suppresses bodily functions such as digestion. The reason for this is that these are non-essential processes in times of emergency, and they are therefore shut down or slowed down so that your body's energy can be directed to where it's needed more urgently.

When considering the sympathetic nervous system, keep in mind that its main purpose is to protect and preserve you in times of danger by stimulating and activating a large number of responses in a single moment. It is closely associated with the body's natural survival instinct, and its role is to turn you into a "superhuman" with heightened senses and increased strength, so that you can find a way out of difficult or dangerous situations.

The Parasympathetic Nervous System

One of the most important functions of the parasympathetic nervous system is to help your body rest, relax, and digest. The parasympathetic nerves will control energy conservation, and is most closely associated with functions that occur during times when you're relaxed and free of physical, emotional, and mental pressure. Since the sympathetic nervous system suppresses digestion, this is one of the most important functions of the parasympathetic nervous system. When your body is relaxed, parasympathetic nerves will signal the intestines to secrete gastric acid in order to digest your food. They will also cause the muscles in your digestive system to move—a movement known as *peristalsis*—and they will stimulate the necessary water and electrolytes to be transported from other parts of your body to aid this process. These nerves will also stimulate the glands in your mouth to produce the saliva necessary to help digest your food. In addition to digestion, your parasympathetic nervous system is also responsible for making tears to lubricate your eyes and contracting your bladder when you urinate.

Another important function of your parasympathetic nervous system is to regulate sleep: When you are relaxed, your nerves will signal the muscles in your heart and lungs to slow down, and constrict your pupils so that less light enters your retinas. This means less energy is needed to move blood and oxygen to these regions of your body, and it can instead be transferred to your gut and intestines in order to digest your food. This creates an important link between sleep and digestion, and why a healthy metabolism can't be maintained if you don't get enough rest.

The parasympathetic nervous system has an important restorative function for your physical body. When food is digested, the energy in it is released into your digestive system. When this happens, it is the job of your parasympathetic nervous system to process this energy and use it to build and restore tissue, and to eliminate any waste that remains. In addition, when your body is in a state of rest, it's also able to grow, reproduce, and repair any damaged cells. As for your mental capabilities, the calmness brought on by the parasympathetic nervous system is essential for you to process memories, improve your ability to learn and think, and retain new information. It's no secret that we can't function—both physically and mentally—without sleep, and this part of the nervous system is the key to improve our quality of sleep and thereby sharpen our daily performance, and our body's ability to heal.

The vagus nerve is not only the longest nerve, but it also makes up 75% of your parasympathetic nervous system. It moves from your brain through your neck, chest, heart, lungs, abdomen, and digestive system. The nerve controls a large number of bodily functions, which include, but are not limited to: Your heart rate, breathing, immune system, and intestines. Because of this range, it's particularly important for your body's ability to "rest and digest."

While some people consider the sympathetic and parasympathetic nervous systems to be in opposition to each other, their relation to each other is more complex than that. While they seem to work in different directions—since one energizes the body, and the other relaxes it—they complement each other in such a way that the body can remain in a stable state. For instance, when you get up after a period of rest—such as first thing in the morning—your blood pressure would drop too low for you to function, had it not been for the sympathetic nervous system's ability to increase your heart rate to prevent this from happening. Similarly, if you are stressed, your sympathetic nervous system will suppress your digestive system and reduce your appetite; however, as soon as the event causing the stress is over, your parasympathetic nervous system will take over so that your body can refuel itself. The human body can't maintain a single state indefinitely—we need periods of rest and of activity, depending on our circumstances—and it's the role of these two nervous systems to make sure there is a balance between these different states. This balance is known as *homeostasis*.

Groundbreaking research—which is discussed in more detail in Chapter 3—proposes that there are three branches of the ANS instead of two. These three works together and they can dial up or down depending on the situation a person finds themselves in; all three are connected by the vagus nerve. The most primitive, the dorsal vagal complex, is activated when confronted by a life-threatening situation, which causes the system to freeze or shut down. The sympathetic nervous system mobilizes the body into fight-or-flight mode, and the ventral vagal complex slows the heart rate and supports a more social state that creates a feeling of safety.

The Autonomic Body

The Regulated and Dysregulated System

Autonomic means "automatic," so in a healthy body with a well-functioning nervous system, there are many functions that should occur without any conscious effort from you. In addition, these functions should be balanced between rest and activity in order to maintain homeostasis in the body. The well-regulated autonomic body is one that is not overwhelmed by stress, and is able to sleep well and rest easily when the time is right. It has a regular digestive system and a well-functioning metabolism, normal blood pressure and a healthy heart. Additionally, it has a strong immune system, a regular breathing rate, a good balance of water and electrolytes. When all of these functions are in place, your autonomic nervous system is in a *regulated state*, which means your body can function efficiently and effectively—as it was made to do.

Autonomic disorders are diseases and illnesses that cause damage to the autonomic nerves. Because nerves play such an important role in the overall functioning of the body, any damage or deterioration of your nerves can have serious consequences. An injured or damaged nerve is one that can't send messages anymore; as a consequence, any functions that this nerve was responsible for will be shut down. For instance, if the sensory nerves in your hands have become damaged, you might experience numbness or tingling when you touch something, or you may have difficulty moving your hands and fingers in a certain way. A body in which the ANS has become damaged in some way can be thought of to be in a *dysregulated state*.

The simplest way in which nerves can become damaged is through physical injury, when they are stretched, crushed, or severed during an accident. Nerve damage can also occur if their blood flow is cut off—for instance, if they are pinched by another part of your body, such as your spine or a tumor, or if a blood vessel becomes blocked before a stroke or heart attack. In addition, they can also become damaged by overuse, as is the case with someone who has carpal tunnel syndrome. Diseases such as cancers, diabetes, lupus, arthritis, infections, and autoimmune diseases, as well as viruses, can also injure nerves. Additionally, there are also certain substances—chemotherapy, poisons, illegal drugs, and excessive amounts of alcohol—that can cause nerve damage.

Unfortunately, nerves also deteriorate with age, and the signals sent by your neurons may become slower over time. It's therefore very important to take care of your nerves, because without them, your body has no way to communicate with itself or the outside world. Accidents can't be prevented, and we're all destined to grow old, so it's impossible to avoid all types of nerve damage. However, if you lead a healthy lifestyle by eating well, getting enough exercise, maintaining good sleep hygiene, regulating stress, and managing any diseases you may have, you can limit nerve damage and improve your body's longevity.

A few common causes of autonomic disorders include Parkinson's disease, diabetes, and aging. However, these disorders can also be caused by more common causes of nerve damage, such as the ones mentioned above. Given the extent to which the ANS regulates the body, there are a vast number of symptoms that can result as a result of autonomic disorders. These include:

- light-headedness as a result of very low blood pressure

- dizziness

- problems urinating, including involuntary urination or difficulty urinating

- constipation

- loss of control over bowel movements

- vomiting

- irritable bowel syndrome and irritable bowel disorder

- a decrease in sweat production

- inability to feel temperature

- dry eyes

- dry mouth

- inability of the pupils to dilate and constrict when the light changes

Always keep in mind that while these symptoms can be a result of damage to the ANS, it's not necessarily always the case. Instead of self-diagnosis, it's better to consult a doctor, especially if these symptoms are very severe, or if they continue to be a problem for long periods of time.

Dysregulation and Mental Health

While autonomic disorders have many physical symptoms, a dysregulated autonomic state also has many consequences for our mental and psychological health. The sympathetic nervous system is activated whenever your body is under stress—and this includes emotional stress. If there is anything in your environment that causes you to become anxious, your sympathetic nervous system will respond by increasing your heart rate and breathing rate, suppressing your appetite, flushing your skin or making you break out in a cold sweat, and possibly causing diarrhea or constipation. At the same time, stress also deactivates your parasympathetic nervous system, which means the nerves that are normally responsible for relaxing your body and returning it to a state of homeostasis can no longer function. Consequently, you become unable to return to a state of rest, and it's for this reason many of us feel stressed for long periods of time with no ability to relax, even when we ought to.

But what does this mean for our mental health? Our brains are an essential part of our nervous system, and they are therefore impacted by any changes or problems we experience as a result of nervous disorders. The nervous system is what connects our brain to many parts of our body, and therefore our physical and mental states can't be separated from each other. A stressed, anxious body with a pounding heart and irregular breathing will result in dysfunctional cognitive abilities, and vice versa. If your body is in this state for too long, it can put too much pressure on your organs, including your brain. Therefore, if your physical health is out of balance, your mental health will be too—and the vagus nerve is central to all of this.

The Vagus Nerve and Mental Imbalances

The Physical Body and Emotional Responses

Your vagus nerve is the "superhighway" of the body, and if it's unhealthy, the rest of your body will be, too. The parasympathetic nervous system can't function when the sympathetic nervous system is activated, which means a body that is in fight-or-flight mode can't experience any rest. Given the size and importance of your vagus nerve, it is therefore this nerve in particular that is suppressed the most during stressful times.

Constant stress has certain physical effects. If these effects continue for too long, you will find yourself flooded by negative emotions and emotional turmoil, as well as the mental imbalances that have come to characterize our modern-day society. Just imagine, for a moment, the effect of being worried or tense for too long: When your heart starts pounding and your breathing becomes too fast, you instantly feel the need to lash out or isolate yourself from others. Sleeping becomes difficult, which leads to chronic fatigue. You may become too overwhelmed to get anything done, your productivity decreases, and your ability to make good decisions becomes impaired. Time management becomes difficult, and you may find yourself procrastinating while all of your focus and energy turns to your stress and anxiety. Your memory may become impaired, and you could find yourself struggling to think, focus, or access previously learned information. You may feel nauseous, your appetite can disappear, or you can find yourself eating too much. You may start catastrophizing your circumstances, or you can find yourself with a restless and unsettled "monkey mind" that only focuses on the negativity and a sense of impending doom. You may start doubting yourself and experience feelings of low self-esteem, or your confidence can suddenly disappear, leaving you anxious, depressed, and stressed all the time. There is more, and unfortunately, all of it can lead to more stress. Before long, you can find yourself in a vicious cycle that can only end in suffering.

In addition to breathing, heart rate, and digestion, your vagus nerve also influences your immune system. As a result, a dysregulated vagus nerve can suppress its ability to control inflammation, which can in turn cause illnesses and diseases. While the occasional cold is normal, constantly feeling unwell will not only impact your everyday functioning, but it can also have an impact on your mood and emotional responses. If this condition persists for too long, it can also lead to mental imbalances.

Another factor that should be considered is the *plasticity* of your brain: If you repeat certain patterns often enough, your brain will change and adapt—or "rewire"—itself according to its circumstances. For instance, if you are constantly negative, your brain will shift itself to this mental state, and repeat it over and over again. Conversely, if you have a positive mindset, the same thing will happen, albeit in reverse. The same goes for a state of worry and stress: If you maintain this state for long enough, it will become your brain and body's default, and it will become more difficult to free yourself from the vicious cycle of mental imbalances. Neuroplasticity is one of our brain's truly remarkable abilities, but it can impede us greatly if we're not careful. On the other hand, we can also harness this great power that we all have to learn how to self-regulate and manage—or even heal—the symptoms we have as a result of dysregulated nervous systems.

The Gut-Brain Axis

Your vagus nerve is closely associated with both your digestive tract and your brain. This connection between these two organs is what is known as the *gut-brain axis*. It might seem unlikely, but think of the butterflies you feel when you think of certain things, or the "gut feeling" you sometimes get. Moreover, certain foods can stimulate brain activity, while others can lower your energy levels and make it difficult to focus. It's clear that your gut and brain are linked, and this connection is facilitated by the vagus nerve.

There are 500 million neurons in your gut, and most of them are connected to your vagus nerve. Just imagine, then what happens to your digestive system—and as a result, your brain—if this nerve becomes suppressed for too long. Constipation, diarrhea, gastrointestinal problems, nausea, vomiting, a slow metabolism, an increased or decreased appetite, and even cravings for certain foods are all associated with an inhibited vagus nerve. While this in itself is a problem, the impact this has on your mental health is even worse. According to Synctuition (2020), "A healthy body is a healthy mind." Therefore, if you're constantly feeling unwell, it's doubtless this will cause or worsen mental imbalances. It is for this reason that a healthy lifestyle and good nutrition is extremely important when it comes to both your body's overall functioning, and your vagus nerve's ability to help you "rest and digest."

Given the state of our society, many of us live in a constant state of stress. This has a severe impact on our vagus nerve, which can in turn harm our mental, physical, and emotional health. The good news is that there's a way out. Your vagus nerve is responsible for calming your body down, so if you learn to activate it, you can access its healing properties and start to manage these mental imbalances that inhibit our day-to-day functioning.

Chapter 3:

Polyvagal Theory

In the past, our understanding of the physical body and emotional and mental health were generally considered separate from each other. However, with the dawn of polyvagal theory, this idea has become the backbone of scientific, medical, and holistic understandings of nervous system dysregulation and its relationship to mental imbalance. There is a strong connection between the sympathetic nervous system, the vagus nerve, and a body that's in a state of dysregulation. This chapter aims to explain why this is the case by describing the following:

- The who, what, and why of polyvagal theory.

- The different states described by polyvagal theory, and what this means for the physical body.

- The role of the vagus nerve in polyvagal theory.

Polyvagal theory has had profound impacts on how we understand our responses to stress. As a type of intersection between neurology and psychology, it can be a way for us to view mental imbalances from a physiological perspective, rather than a purely psychological one. More specifically, it teaches us how our vagus nerve causes interactions in our physical body that can have enormous effects on our mental and emotional health.

What Is Polyvagal Theory?

The Different Neural Circuits of Polyvagal Theory

On the 8th of October, 1994, Dr. Stephen W. Porges astounded the Society of Psychophysiological Research during his presidential address. For some years, he had studied the way in which our bodies process stress. In his address, he proposed that our nervous system is closely connected to how our bodies react to stress, and that this affects our emotional and mental states. Before Porges' theory, it was believed that your body had only two states when it came to stress. You were either stressed, or you weren't, and you could shift from one to the other by eliminating the stressor. In primitive human societies, this type of response makes sense: People were threatened or attacked by something in their natural environment, which caused them to react with a stress response from their sympathetic nervous system. However, the stressor—whether it be a predator, natural disaster, or strife amongst their peers, would inevitably be removed again, which would allow the person to return to an unstressed state in which their parasympathetic nervous systems could be activated.

In this understanding of the human stress response, there was no space for any in-between states or different levels of being stressed. In addition, it didn't account for the consequences of prolonged pressure, such as those that we experience in our modern-day lives. As a result, many of the therapies developed to reduce stress aimed to "switch off" the stressed state to return the body to a place where it wasn't under pressure. While these therapies did work for some people—and continue to do so—the state of the global population's mental health is evidence that they are not, in fact, as effective as we need them to be.

According to Dr. Porges, there are three neural circuits of the vagus nerve, namely the *ventral*, the *sympathetic*, and the *dorsal* states. The social engagement circuit, or *ventral vagal* pathway, is reached when the nervous system is calm and relaxed. This circuit encourages a more social state with those feelings of connection and safety that are so important to human beings. The ventral state is more conducive to accurately interpreting facial expressions and body language. When this circuit is activated, we can feel empathy and we have access to emotions such as happiness, love, and joy. This translates into feelings of safety and security, which has a positive impact on our overall well-being and our ability to remain present in the moment. This is also the state in which the body can heal and rejuvenate itself.

Fight or flight, or *sympathetic reaction* to mobilize, is the state our bodies turn to when we become stressed. This neural circuit is closely associated with human beings' natural survival instinct, and serves the purpose of forcing us into action so that we can protect ourselves from danger. In the modern world, this fight-or-flight action might look like the decision to confront a nagging boss, trying to meet a deadline, or running away after being mugged in the subway. The problem is that these modern stressors don't always go away: The nagging boss might still be in your life, your job likely has an endless stream of deadlines, and you still have to take the subway home after work every day. Sympathetic activation causes many physiological responses such as a raised heart rate, high blood pressure, suppression of the immune system, and the release of cortisol in the body. If, because of chronic stress, your nervous system is never allowed to re-regulate itself after an event, it can become the root of chronic illness—and this is where anxiety lives.

Immobilization, or the *dorsal vagus response* is the third neural circuit, and it kicks in after receiving cues that the body is in life-threatening danger. It moves us away from a state of connection into one of protection. When this circuit becomes activated, we shift into immobilization; this can be seen as freezing, blanking out, shutting down, or disassociating. In animals, we see this when they decide to "play dead"—it means the danger they experience has shifted them into a "freeze" state. When this happens, all bodily functions shut down and only emergency life support systems continue to run in the background.

We move between each of these states throughout the day, and it's normal to experience them all in a short period of time. The three circuits actually work together, and they continuously turn up or turn down as the system tries to re-regulate itself. For example, you can be socially engaged while still experiencing some stress, or you can be despondent but still have bursts of adrenaline from momentary sympathetic activation.

Polyvagal Theory in the Human Body and Mind

The sympathetic activation and dorsal vagal states are both relatively primitive neural circuits, and are therefore closely associated with our natural survival instinct. The reason why our bodies move into these states is because it's trying to protect and preserve itself. Being in survival mode has remarkable effects on our bodies, but it also has several cognitive consequences. One of these is how we make sense of reality. When we move into states of sympathetic activation or dorsal vagal shutdown, our perception of the world around us changes. Instead of seeing things for what they are, we actually come to view everything around us as more threatening. While this is partly a mental construct, it has been proven to show up in physiological ways, too. For instance, your hearing will shift so that you are more prone to hear low-frequency sounds, such as those our ancestors associated with the growls of predators. Neutral facial expressions can seem more aggressive, or fear in others can be interpreted as anger. As a result, it becomes difficult to interpret other people's intent or behavior. Humans use dozens of cues, sometimes subconsciously, to determine how safe a situation is and how to feel, and the body responds in kind. Dr. Porges calls this *neuroception.*

Being unable to self-regulate makes life difficult, and the constant effort of trying to keep ourselves afloat in a threatening environment—while at the same time trying to manage our emotions despite our tension and fear—saps the energy out of us. This decreases our performance, which in turn leads to more stress, which reactivates our sympathetic nervous system—and so the cycle continues. Being caught up in this cycle also means that your body never gets the rest it needs, and your cells are never able to fully regenerate and recover. Feeling fatigued and physically unwell has consequences for your cognitive functioning and your relationships. As a result, your physical and mental health will suffer.

Polyvagal theory has had a profound impact on how we understand ourselves, because it combines neurology and psychology to give a physiological explanation of our behavior. Simply put, our nervous systems pick up signs in the environment, and evaluate them on a subconscious level. When these signs seem dangerous in any way, our neural circuits respond by activating and deactivating certain parts of our bodies. This, in turn, changes how we relate to the world, which then has an impact on how we react to things around us. Thus, our behavior and emotional responses are not isolated to our brains alone—they are also the product of a complex series of processes that happen within our physical bodies. It's important to remember that the signs our bodies respond to might not even be overtly threatening.

Chapter 4:

Signs of a Dysfunctional Vagus

Nerve

Your vagus nerve is connected to a number of important organs and functions in your body. For this reason, a dysfunctional vagus nerve can cause many serious health issues. On the other hand, if you understand how this nerve works relative to the rest of your body, it can also start to function as an "early-warning system" to help you identify problems in your physical, mental, and emotional health before they start to interfere with your life. This chapter looks at the following:

- What it means when your vagus nerve is dysfunctional, and what some of the causes are of vagal nerve dysfunction.

- The three types of pain you can experience.

- The physiological and psychological symptoms that show up if your vagus nerve is dysfunctional.

- Where in your body you can expect to experience pain as a result of a dysfunctional vagus nerve.

While the vagus nerve is an important part of your body, there are many other organs, glands, and nerves that can also cause you to experience uncomfortable or painful physiological and psychological symptoms. That being said, combining your understanding of the role of the vagus nerve in the nervous system with the ideas proposed by polyvagal theory can provide you with a powerful tool to identify and relieve a large number of health issues. After all, the vagus nerve is your body's superpower!

Your Body Doesn't Lie

The human body is an extremely complex system made up of billions of different parts, and if even one of these parts are dysfunctional, it will show up in one way or another. The human body doesn't lie—if it causes you to experience any unusual or uncomfortable symptoms, it always means there is something wrong. This is good news for those who are willing to listen because it means you can resolve many health issues, by simply paying attention. The vagus nerve in particular is a powerful tool because of its extensive reach within the body. If you are willing to pay attention to it, you'll be able to harness its incredible power in your life.

Vagal nerve dysfunction is serious business—but what does *dysfunctional* mean in your nervous system? Generally, speaking, something that is dysfunctional is not working as it should. In technology, it means your electrical device is faulty, and in social situations, it means there are problems in your relationship. In the human body, a dysfunctional vagus nerve means it's not regulating all the different parts as it should.

Vagal nerve dysfunction can be the result of a number of things. Because it is a nerve, it's subject to the same injuries and damage other nerves can suffer, as seen in Chapter 2. There are, however, a few causes of vagal nerve dysfunction that are far more prevalent than others. Some of these are stress, fear, and unending tension. As seen before, if your body catches even the slightest whiff of danger—and this includes emotional and mental pressure, as well as physical strain—it will activate your sympathetic nervous system in order to help you escape the circumstances that are causing you stress. In a primitive society where danger could be easily escaped, this was a fairly useful response to fear. However, in our modern lives there is simply too much pressure to escape, which means our sympathetic nervous system is activated constantly.

Your vagus nerve can also become overstimulated, which will cause the heart to slow down and blood vessels in your body—especially the lower body—to dilate. In turn, the blood flow in your body changes, and the brain is deprived of oxygen; this can cause you to lose consciousness. This is what's known as a *vagal response* or *vasovagal reflex*, and it can lead to uncomfortable, painful, or even dangerous symptoms. It's also a sign of a dysfunctional vagus nerve.

Another way to describe the efficiency of the vagus nerve is through *vagal tone*. This is a measurement of how effectively your vagus nerve responds to certain situations, and how quickly you return to homeostasis. If you have a high vagal tone, it means your physical body—especially your heart, lungs, and gut—is healthy, and that you're able to regulate your emotions and your stress responses. The time it takes you to relax after a stressful event is also an indication of your vagal tone. Therefore, someone who can calm themselves easily, can be considered to have a healthy vagus nerve. On the other hand, a low vagal tone is associated with poor health and an inability to regulate. There are several different ways to test your vagal tone, and these are described in Chapter 5. *Toning* your vagal nerve means improving its functioning through certain exercises and practices which are discussed in Chapter 7, 8, and 9. If you currently have a low vagal tone, there are ways to improve it so that you can live a fuller and healthier life.

The Body's Messages

Your body—and in particular, your vagus nerve—is an amazing organism that will tell you if something is wrong. However, it's no use committing yourself to listening to its messages if you don't understand what they mean. Oftentimes, any problems in the body show up as some sort of pain. We tend to pay the most attention to physical pain, as this is the easiest to describe. Dysfunction in your body can also show up as mental or emotional pain.

There are thousands of different types of pain we can experience, and some of them you may never even have heard of. To make it easier to identify and understand your body, the different types of pain have been divided into three categories: Structural, chemical, and neurological pain.

Structural Pain

The structure of something is a description of its sturdiness and strength… So yes, you guessed it: Structural pain is related to your physical body. More specifically, it refers to any injuries you may have suffered, or physical imbalances you experience. If you twist your ankle or break your arm, for instance, you'll experience structural pain in those parts of your body. In addition, any other physical pain—such as stomach cramps, difficulty breathing, or problems with your heart rate—are also considered structural, even though it's not the result of obvious external injury.

The vagus nerve can cause many types of structural pain, most of which can be felt in your head, chest or abdomen. However, a dysfunctional vagus nerve can also lead to discomfort in parts of your back, hands and feet, as well as joints. If your vagus nerve becomes dysregulated in this way, it means it's trying to warn you to change something in your life, so that you can begin to heal yourself.

Chemical Pain

Nerves are what connects the different parts of your body to each other, and communicate through chemical transmission. There are many ways in which your nerves can become injured, and one of these is through damage to its transmission system. In addition, your sympathetic and parasympathetic nervous systems also sometimes join forces with your enteric nervous system, which is the part of your body that's responsible for releasing and regulating chemicals such as hormones. Any dysfunction in these parts of your body can therefore cause pain of a chemical nature.

Chemical pain can show up in a number of ways, but the most common are chronic stress, inflammation, physiological pain, mental stress, and emotional dysfunction. For instance, chronic stress can be the result of your body releasing a hormone known as cortisol, which is also known as the "stress hormone." Inflammation typically occurs when your body's immune system becomes compromised or attacked in some way, or if you suffer some sort of physical damage to your body. In response to the attack or the damage, your nervous system signals your body to release cells to the site of the damage in order to fight off the pathogen or heal the injury. Sometimes, however, your body can release these cells to a place where there is nothing to fight off, and this causes inflammation to occur. As for mental stress and emotional dysfunction, these can be caused by any number of things, including a dysregulated autonomic nervous system, chemicals in your brain that are out of balance, or hormones in your body that are not well-regulated.

Neurological Pain

Neurological pain is related to your brain and your nervous system, and typically shows up as chronic stress or pain in your head and facial region, such as headaches. There are many types of headaches, including tension headaches, sinus headaches, cluster headaches, migraines, or hormone headaches. These can occur in different parts of your brain, and the trick to diagnosing them is normally to try and identify which part of your head hurts. For example, a sinus headache will cause pain in the front part of your head around your forehead, cheekbones, and nose, while a cluster headache will cause pain around your eye.

There is some overlap between the different types of pain; for instance, the symptoms of stress are both chemical and neurological, and the pain caused by inflammation can be both structural and chemical. The important thing, however, is not to be able to categorize the pain you're feeling, but rather to know your body well enough to realize you are experiencing pain in the first place. Even if you can't accurately identify what it is that is causing your suffering, it's still important to acknowledge it, and to treat it as soon as you notice it's there. Dealing with symptoms can be scary, but keep in mind that anything that's ignored for too long will only get worse. The sooner you respond to pain, the sooner you can heal—and that's why it's important to listen to your body.

Physiological Symptoms of Vagal Nerve Dysfunction

A dysfunctional nerve nerve—whether it be over- or under-stimulated—can cause a variety of symptoms. Your vagus nerve connects to many different parts of your body, which means these symptoms can occur all over your body. In addition, your vagus nerve can result in many different types of pain, including structural, chemical, and neurological discomfort. The list is nearly endless, but below are some of the common physical symptoms of a dysregulated vagus nerve, and how it might feel.

Headaches, Ear Pain, and Neck Pain

The neck moves constantly, while at the same time, serves as a pathway for the vagal nerves that originate in the brain. It's therefore very possible for the vagus nerve to become irritated or injured as a result of this movement. For example, if the nerves are pinched by the spine, the resulting blood loss to the nerve can cause it to become dysfunctional. Similarly, poor posture can also cut off or reduce the vagus nerve's blood supply, with a number of consequences, such as headaches. Headaches can take on many forms, and they can occur in different parts of the brain. Oftentimes, they result from certain chemical activity in your brain, or if the blood vessels in your skull are dysfunctional. They can also result from injury to the muscles in your neck and head. The vagus nerve's function in this regard is to regulate the signals sent to muscles and blood vessels. In addition, the vagus nerve is also in control of the pain pathways that lead to the brain, and stimulating it can therefore change our brain's response to pain.

Neck pain can also lead to a dysfunctional vagus nerve, especially if the pain is accompanied by tight muscles in this area, such as the SCM muscle. Tightness in this area will put pressure on the vagus nerve, which in turn can lead to dysregulation. Exercises to lengthen and release this muscle are described in Chapter 8. Depending on the severity of the vagal nerve dysfunction, headaches and neck pain can be intense, and even chronic. Studies have also shown that chronic pain can lead to depression and anxiety, which is further proof of the vagus nerve's impact on both physical and emotional health.

Dizziness and Light-Headedness

A vagal response will cause more blood to flow into your lower body, which will in turn deprive your brain of blood and oxygen. As a result, you can begin to feel dizzy or light-headed. In severe cases, this sudden drop in blood pressure can make you faint; this is known as *vasovagal syncope*. Feeling dizzy is not only uncomfortable, but it can also be dangerous. Your brain needs oxygen in order to function, and if it's deprived of this for too long, the consequences can be quite severe.

Blurred Vision or Tunnel Vision

Sometimes people have an overreaction to a situation—such as fear or the sight of blood—which can trigger a vasovagal response. This response causes the person's blood pressure and heart rate to drop suddenly, which reduces blood flow to the brain and bodily functions located in the head. As a result, you can feel dizzy, faint, or have blurred or tunnel vision.

Ringing Ears and Tinnitus

Tinnitus is a condition in which someone experiences constant ringing in one or both of their ears. This sound can also present itself as buzzing, clicking, humming, hissing, or roaring, and it originates within the ear. It's a disorder that can be chronic—and therefore extremely disruptive—and is generally associated with old-age. However, that's not always the case: A dysfunctional vagus nerve can also lie at the root of this problem.

There are many possible causes of tinnitus. One of these is that changes in the brain can adjust the signals sent to your auditory system by your nerves, which can affect your hearing. More specifically, it's believed tinnitus is caused by increased neural activity as a result of injury to the head, auditory canals, or blood vessels in this region. There are many nerves involved in your hearing, but one of the most important is the vagus nerve. By re-regulating the vagus nerve, it can rewire the signals sent by the brain to the ears and cause the brain to adapt in such a way that the ringing stops. Studies are currently being conducted to investigate *VNS*—vagus nerve stimulator that is implanted in the body—to see if they can lead to any significant improvements for patients.

A vasovagal response can also cause your ears to ring as a result of sudden reduced blood flow to the brain. This type of response is normally accompanied by nausea and dizziness, and a lot of people have reported feeling this just before fainting. This can be a sign that the body is having a dorsal vagal response, and it's usually temporary. However, if this happens frequently, it can be a sign of vagal dysregulation.

Clenched Teeth, Jaw Pain, Bruxism, and TMJ Disorders

There is increasing research into the link between low vagal tone, clenched teeth, and jaw pain. Discomfort in this region is often associated with strain in the muscles and joints that are responsible for moving the jaw, and it can take on several forms. One of these is *bruxism*, which is the unconscious, excessive grinding and clenching of your teeth. Another is *temporomandibular*—or TMJ—disorders, which occur when the joint connecting your jawbone to your skull becomes damaged. These disorders have a number of symptoms, one of the most common being a "clicking" sound in your jaw whenever you use your jaw. Other symptoms include pain in your jaw or around your ears, difficulty chewing, and a locked joint that can prevent you from opening or closing your mouth.

While clenched teeth and jaw pain are physiological symptoms, there are a lot of studies that indicate these are closely associated with our mental and emotional health. There is an especially important relationship between stress, fatigue, anxiety—all of which are associated with a dysregulated nervous system—and bruxism and TMJ disorders. Activation of the sympathetic nervous system causes our muscles to tense, which includes the muscles in our jaws. In someone with low vagal tone, it can be difficult, or even impossible, to relax these muscles, which means the joints that connect your muscles, skull, and jaw become worn out. One possible treatment is to re-regulate the vagus nerve.

Coughing, Difficulty Swallowing, and Vocal Hoarseness

One of the vagus nerve's biggest motor functions is to control the muscles in your throat. This muscle is responsible for your ability to swallow, your gag reflex, and the vibration of your vocal cords to produce sounds. For instance, there are reflexive muscles in your throat that prevent food you're swallowing from moving into your airway while you're eating. Injury to the vagus nerve in this area can therefore cause these muscles to become dysfunctional. Possible symptoms include difficulty swallowing and the loss of your gag reflex, constant coughing, or changes to the vocal cord, such as tremors, hoarseness, wheezing, or the complete loss of your voice. A good way to start healing this is by toning the vagus nerve.

Thyroid Disorders

Your thyroid is a gland that produces the hormones your body needs to control your heart rate, body temperature, blood pressure, and weight. It is located at the base of your throat, and it's activated by the vagus nerve. If this nerve is damaged or dysfunctional, it can cause many problems throughout your body. For instance, an underactive thyroid—also known as *hypothyroidism*—causes weight gain, joint pain, fatigue, and muscle weakness. Your thyroid also controls your body's responses to temperature, so someone whose gland is overactive can find themselves becoming more sensitive to cold—particularly in their hands and feet—or more prone to excessive sweating. Their skin can become drier or puffier— especially in the facial region—and the risk for heart disease, an elevated heart rate and blood pressure, and increased cholesterol levels becomes greater.

On the other hand, *hyperthyroidism*, which is an overactive thyroid, can cause just as many health problems: Unintentional and rapid weight loss, a rapid or irregular heartbeat, heart palpitations, trembling hands and fingers, excessive sweating, thinning and drying skin, and an increased sensitivity to heat are all caused by this disorder, and they can be just as severe as hypothyroidism.

Interestingly, the reach of your thyroid is so extensive that it can even lead to thinning or loss of hair if it becomes under- or overactive. Hyper- and hypothyroidism also has certain psychological symptoms; some of these include insomnia, difficulty remembering, difficulty concentrating, anxiety and irritability, and depression. These symptoms may take some time to develop, but if they do, they can severely disrupt your life. Thyroid disorders are very complex and can arise as a result of a number of reasons, some of which are connected to the vagus nerve. You should consult a doctor if you are having thyroid issues, as there are important medications for this disorder. Using traditional medical therapies in conjunction with toning the vagus nerve can be beneficial.

Muscle Tension

Pain in the muscles can become so severe, it can prevent someone from being able to walk. Your vagus nerve is responsible for stimulating many muscles in your body, so if it becomes inflamed, it can lead to cramps and tension that may or may not be chronic. Vagus-related muscle pain is especially prevalent in the back, shoulders, and neck, and it can be released by performing some of the exercises described in Chapters 7, 8, and 9.

High and Low Blood Pressure

The vagus nerve can be dysfunctional in more than one way, which means it can cause seemingly contradicting symptoms. If your vagus nerve is suppressed or you have a low vagal tone—especially as a result of an overactive sympathetic nervous system—your heart will beat too fast, which will result in high blood pressure, or *hypertension*. This can also be accompanied by an increased breathing rate, and can result in feelings of stress and anxiety. Chronic high blood pressure over a long period of time can damage your arteries and put too much pressure on your heart, which in turn can lead to diseases such as heart attacks and chest pain.

In contrast, if your vagus nerve is overactive, your heart will beat too slowly and cause low blood pressure, or *hypotension*. As a consequence, you may feel dizzy if you stand up too quickly, or you may suffer from occasional fainting spells. Low blood pressure is also associated with tiredness, nausea, ringing ears, and blurred vision.

Breathing Difficulties and Asthma

The vagus nerve is responsible for a lot of the movement in our lungs, which means neural dysfunction can lead to breathing-related problems. Damage to the vagus nerve in this area can make it feel as if your breath is obstructed, or you can suffer from uncontrollable and constant hiccupping. *Asthma* is a condition of the lungs that arises when vessels in these organs become constricted. The vagus nerve is responsible for the dilation or constriction of these vessels, which means stimulating it can have many benefits for managing the symptoms associated with asthma and other breathing difficulties.

Gastrointestinal Issues and Gastroparesis

Your vagus nerve is connected to your stomach and intestines, which means any vagal dysfunction can cause problems in these areas. If your vagus nerve is underactive or inactive as a result of a low vagal tone, the digestive system may become suppressed: It will release too few or too many digestive enzymes. Furthermore, the level of acidity in the stomach can become imbalanced, and the muscles in the digestive tract can become inactive or start to contract involuntarily. As a result, food will move through the digestive tract too slowly, which means it will stay in the system for too long. This can have a variety of consequences, including nausea and vomiting, indigestion, acid reflux, low appetite, weight loss, bloating, erratic changes in your blood sugar levels, and stomach aches. These symptoms can occur on their own or in conjunction with each other. They can also be indicators of a vagal-nerve-related condition in the digestive tract known as *gastroparesis*, although this isn't always the case.

In addition to gastroparesis, a dysfunctional vagus nerve can also cause other gut-related symptoms, such as nutrient deficiencies, irritable bowel syndrome, Crohn's Disease, insulin dysregulation, and stomach ulcers.

Nutrient Deficiencies

The vagus nerve stimulates cells in the stomach to secrete the necessary chemicals to absorb certain nutrients. If your vagus nerve is underactive, the levels in which these chemicals occur won't be right, which in turn means the nutrients in your food are not broken down and absorbed as they would be in a person with a functional vagus nerve. Vitamin B12 deficiencies are especially related to vagal nerve dysfunction.

Nutrient deficiencies can have severe consequences. In the case of vitamin B12, not getting enough of this substance in your body can result in further nerve damage, dementia, or even death.

Irritable Bowel Syndrome (IBS), Irritable Bowel Disorder (IBD), and Crohn's Disease

IBS and IBD are two diseases of the intestines that can have uncomfortable or painful symptoms, depending on their severity. Some of these include abdominal pain or stomach cramps, bloating, constipation or diarrhea—or a combination of both—and flatulence. Like IBS and IBD, Crohn's disease is caused by inflammation in the digestive tract, although its symptoms may be more severe. The vagus nerve is an important source of control in the body's immune system, and it's responsible for preventing inflammation from occurring. This means a dysfunctional vagus nerve will be unable to prevent the body from attacking its own cells, and the resulting inflammation can cause severe pain and discomfort.

Insulin Dysregulation and Weight Gain

The vagus nerve is responsible for keeping the body in homeostasis by regulating glucose production and insulin secretion. Both of these chemicals are essential in the way your body processes nutrients. As a result, a dysfunctional vagus nerve can lead to changes in appetite and weight. In severe cases, vagal dysregulation has also been connected to diabetes, which is a disease that occurs in people whose bodies don't produce the insulin necessary to regulate their blood sugar levels.

Stomach Ulcers

Stomach ulcers are sores that develop on the insides of your stomach lining and intestines as a result of these linings releasing too much acid. Ulcers can be extremely painful, and they present themselves as stomach pain, bloating, a burning sensation in the stomach, or discomfort when eating or drinking. Your stomach has to produce and release acid in order to help digest your food. However, if your vagus nerve is dysfunctional, the amount of acid released won't be regulated well, and this can burn the inside of the stomach and intestines.

Lowered Immunity and Chronic Inflammation

The purpose of your immune system is to fight off any foreign bodies or pathogens—known as *antigens*—that enter your body, and it does this by making and releasing antibodies whenever it detects any of these antigens. The immune system is part of the ANS, and the vagus nerve plays a large role in the immune response. If a vagus nerve is dysfunctional, your body's natural response to antigens can become impaired and it won't be able to fight off diseases very easily, which means you will become ill easier and more often.

In addition to illness, a further consequence of an ineffective immune system is inflammation. This occurs when the body starts attacking its own cells because it considers these to be foreign. There are a large number of diseases and disorders that are associated with inflammation, including sepsis, arthritis, multiple sclerosis, Alzheimer's disease, and inflammatory bowel disease. The purpose of the vagus nerve is to signal to the brain to suppress the cells that cause inflammation in our bodies. If it has become dysregulated, however, the communication between the nervous system and the brain won't be as efficient as it needs to be, and this can arise in the form of inflammatory symptoms.

Psychological Symptoms of Vagal Nerve Dysfunction

Your brain is the source of your mental and emotional activity; it is also the place where your vagus nerve starts its journey. In addition to the problems that arise as a direct relationship between your vagus nerve and your brain, the physical symptoms caused by a dysregulated nervous system—especially if they're chronic—can also cause mental and emotional stress. For example, being in constant pain can lead to frustration, depression, irritability, or anger.

It has been proven before that there is a relationship between your body and your brain. As a result, dysfunction in your mental and emotional health doesn't always present itself as psychological disorders. Instead, these can also show up in the form of physiological symptoms. Furthermore, psychological symptoms often cause us to feel certain physical sensations: Anxiety can cause your stomach to flutter or your spine to tingle, while anger and sadness can make your chest feel tight and constricted. The key to understanding your psychological symptoms is to identify where in your body you feel them. This is why it's important to cultivate an awareness of both your emotional responses as well as your physical body, and to understand how these two are related to each other. Healing yourself successfully means listening, understanding, and finally, acting.

Despondence, Hopelessness, and Helplessness

When your system goes into dorsal vagal shutdown, one of the symptoms you may experience are feelings of hopelessness and despondency. It may seem as though you've lost all agency and are incapable of making decisions on your own. In addition, you may also feel helpless because you're unable to see your way out of your present circumstances. This happens because your body has become so tired that it has decided to simply shut down in order to restore homeostasis and allow your system an opportunity to rest. In addition to the emotional distress caused by dorsal vagal shutdown, you can also experience it physically in the form of a "heaviness" that spreads throughout your body.

Anger

Anger is a feeling we all experience occasionally, but if it's chronic and uncontrollable, it can also be a sign that something is wrong in your body. Anger is typically triggered by an external factor, such as things that make us feel attacked or unsafe. Being in fight-or-flight mode is therefore a possible cause of anger. With that being said, a low vagal tone will result in you being unable to revert from that state back into parasympathetic activation. At the same time, our anger can also be triggered when we feel hopeless, powerless, and out of control, which are symptoms that arise very easily when our bodies move into dorsal vagal shutdown. Anger shows up as tightness in the chest or head, and can also cause your skin to become flushed.

Irritability and Frustration

While dorsal vagal shutdown is your body's attempt to restore balance and give you an opportunity to rest; feeling hopeless, tired, and despondent can cause irritability and frustration—especially with ourselves. To make matters worse, if you are having difficulty self-regulating your emotions, these feelings can get out of control and make you lash out at other people in an attempt to express your own personal frustration. Being unable to do the things we need to do can be very annoying, and oftentimes the root of these problems lie in vagus nerve dysfunction.

Sadness and Depression

Sadness and depression are not the same thing, but there is some overlap between the two. *Sadness* is an emotion that we all occasionally feel, and it is triggered by external events. *Depression*, on the other hand, is sadness that has become chronic and persistent, and that doesn't seem to be triggered by anything specific. If your emotions have started impacting your functioning, it might mean they are more than just the average "human experience."

When people become depressed, they feel helpless and listless, and they often have the need to isolate themselves. In contrast with ventral vagal activation that puts us in a state of social engagement, dorsal vagal shutdown is responsible for many of the emotions we associate with depression. Unlike other emotions, depression is not felt physically in any part of the body. Rather, it deactivates your senses so that you may start to feel numb and disconnected—even from yourself.

Lack of Energy and Chronic Fatigue

Low energy levels can show up as the need to sleep constantly, but it can also make you feel as if your entire body is too heavy to move. Being lackluster and lethargic, and unwilling or unable to do anything are all signs of having a lack of energy. Feeling occasional tiredness is normal, especially if you've had a busy day at work or you exercised a lot. However, being lethargic is a problem when it becomes chronic. Being fatigued can make someone want to sleep all the time, or they may find they're not well-rested, even when they do sleep enough. In contrast to the sympathetic nervous system, the vagus nerve lowers your energy levels so that you can go into a state of rest and digest. However, if your vagus nerve is dysfunctional, this can severely limit your day-to-day functioning.

Brain Fog

A dysfunctional vagus nerve can show up as "brain fog," especially when you are very tired. There are a number of symptoms associated with this situation, including poor memory and forgetfulness as well as difficulty concentrating. Researchers are not yet entirely decided on what causes the fatigue that results in brain fog, but one of the theories claims that a dysfunctional vagus nerve will continually signal to the brain to behave as though the body is physically ill. Another theory is that the parasympathetic nervous system constricts blood vessels in some parts of the body when it's activated, which reduces blood and oxygen flow to the brain and creates the sensation of being unable to think clearly. Other potential causes of brain fog include insomnia, depression, and hypothyroidism—all of which can be connected to the vagus nerve.

Worry, Anxiety, and Panic Attacks

Your sympathetic nervous system is what causes you to experience the symptoms—such as a pounding heart and difficulty breathing—typically associated with anxiety, and it's the role of the vagus nerve to counteract these symptoms. However, in the case of vagal dysfunction, there is nothing to counteract the sympathetic nervous system and your stress response can therefore run along unchecked. In very severe cases, feelings of intense anxiety can become so severe that they escalate and peak within a matter of minutes: this is what causes panic attacks. Anxiety can be felt all over the body, but it's most commonly associated with the heart and lungs as well as erratic mental activity.

Restlessness and Racing Thoughts

When the sympathetic nervous system is activated, the body receives a boost of physical and mental energy. This mobilizes you to think more clearly and be more active. However, this same response can also turn into restlessness and racing thoughts, especially if low vagal tone prevents someone from successfully allowing their parasympathetic nervous system to take over and calm them down. These symptoms are also often associated with anxiety, as well as ADD and ADHD, which are discussed below.

Chronic Stress

We will all feel pressure of some sort in our lives, and the occasional feelings of stress and tension are normal. However, stress becomes a problem when it continues for an extended period of time with no or very few breaks in between. People with chronic stress wake up worried and they go to sleep worried—if they sleep at all. This is because their low vagal tone is preventing their parasympathetic nervous systems from becoming activated, and they remain in constant fight-or-flight mode. Chronic stress is associated with a whole host of other symptoms, including insomnia, physical weakness, inability to focus, difficulty socializing, and muscle aches and pains.

Insomnia

Insomnia is what is known as a chronic inability to come to rest, or to fall asleep at night. People with this disorder might also wake up regularly during the night, wake up too early, never go into a state of deep sleep, or still not feel rested even though they've had a full night's sleep. Sleep is vital to our functioning, and having insomnia can give rise to a whole host of other symptoms, such as difficulty regulating your moods, physical illness and weakness, and brain fog. Given the role of the vagus nerve in helping your body to calm itself, it's no surprise that a dysfunctional nerve will inhibit your ability to fall asleep at night, or to stay asleep for long enough for you to get the rest and recovery you need.

Attention Deficit Disorder and Attention Deficit Hyperactivity Disorder

Attention Deficit Disorder (ADD) or *Attention Deficit Hyperactivity Disorder* (ADHD) arise when someone is chronically unable to remain focused or to regulate their emotions. The vagus nerve plays an important part in these disorders because the pathways in the brain that are responsible for our ability to stay alert are affected by stress. If someone has a low vagal tone, the balance between their sympathetic and parasympathetic nervous systems will be impaired, which can cause ADD and ADHD. These disorders have many symptoms, including restlessness, racing thoughts, difficulty concentrating, and becoming distracted easily. In very severe cases, they can greatly affect someone's ability to maintain relationships and jobs.

Epilepsy

There are many studies that show that stimulating the vagus nerve can reduce seizures and epilepsy. There are a few possible reasons for this, but one is that the vagus nerve influences blood flow in the brain, and that a stimulated vagus nerve can therefore activate the inactive parts of the brain that are the cause of seizures. Another theory suggests that seizures can be treated by activating the electrical signals used for communication between the brain and the vagus nerve. There have also been suggestions that the vagus nerve releases certain chemicals into the brain when stimulated which also has an impact on seizures. In patients who are drug resistant, a VNS device—or vagus nerve stimulator—is implanted in the body and attached to the left side of the vagus nerve. The purpose of a VNS is to send regular, gentle, electrical pulses through the vagus nerve to calm the irregular electrical brain activity that may be the cause of seizures.

Eating Problems and Disorders

Your vagus nerve is directly responsible for most of what happens in your gut, including your appetite and metabolism. At the same time, it also controls a lot of your cognitive functioning, including things such as mood and cravings. There is a close association between mental imbalance and appetite. For instance, someone suffering from depression may lose their appetite completely, while people who are stressed have often reported binging or "comfort eating" to get temporary relief from their emotional pain through food. This can lead to rapid weight gain or loss, or even eating disorders. A dysfunctional vagus nerve can also cause physiological symptoms—such as loss of appetite or a slow metabolism—that can also impact metabolism and weight.

Chapter 5:

Testing Your Vagus Nerve

A dysfunctional vagus nerve can be treated, but in order to do so, you first have to know whether or not it requires reregulation. This chapter digs deeper into how this can be done by looking at the following:

- What the natural state of your vagus nerve should be.

- How your vagus nerve can move out of this state by deregulating itself.

- How you can learn to control your vagus nerve.

- Ways to test your vagus nerve so that you can ascertain if it has become dysfunctional or not by looking at the following methods:

    o   facial observation

    o   heart rate variability

    o   pharyngeal ventral branch function

    o   trap squeeze

    o   ventral brake

- What steps should be followed for each method, and how you should interpret the results of your tests.

Your body is a magical set of complex systems that will always tell you if something is wrong or out of balance. If you want to learn to harness one of its biggest superpowers—the vagus nerve—you also have to learn to listen and understand it before you try to respond.

The Natural State

It's normal in any human body for the sympathetic nervous system to become stimulated from time to time. When this happens, the vagus nerve becomes suppressed in a sense—or *deregulated*. This is a normal part of human functioning, and in the right circumstances, it is essential to our survival. At the same time, the vagus nerve has the ability to *re-regulate* itself after a stressful event—and this is where many of our problems lie.

First, let's take a look at how the vagus nerve re-regulates itself. In a healthy body, the parasympathetic nervous system will become activated once a stressful event has passed. This happens because our fight-or-flight response puts strain on our physical and mental functioning, and we therefore need to recover after such an event. The parasympathetic nervous system is stimulated by a safe environment. In other words, as soon as your subconscious mind is assured that you are safe and the danger you were facing is gone, it will trigger your rest and digest response, including your vagus nerve.

Once the vagus nerve is activated, the following happens:

- The nerves in your ears are activated to allow you to feel pressure, temperature, touch, and moisture.

- Your throat muscles become stimulated so that your gag reflex functions normally and you can swallow your food.

- The muscles that control your airways and vocal cords begin to function efficiently, which allows you to speak normally and at your natural pitch.

- Your breathing rate slows down and your breaths become deeper, because your vagus nerve signals the muscles in your airways to open up.

- Your heart muscles are slowed down so that the force with which it's pumping blood is lowered, which in turn reduces your heart rate.

- A combination of your heart rate and your kidney functioning changes the size of your blood vessels to lower your blood pressure.

- The vagus nerve stimulates your digestive system—including the gastric juices and saliva that helps to digest your food—so that any food in your intestines is processed and eliminated, your body can accurately determine whether it's hungry or full.

- Your metabolism is influenced, which signals to your body when insulin should be released into your bloodstream; this in turn has an effect on your blood sugar levels, and therefore the amount of energy you have.

- Your immune system is appropriately activated or deactivated depending on whether there are any pathogens in your body or not.

- New neural connections are formed in your brain, which allows you to absorb new information and form new memories.

Activating your parasympathetic nervous system—and by extension, your vagus nerve—restores the balance in your body and puts it back into a state of homeostasis. Since your body is inclined to always return to a state of balance, it will involuntarily do what needs to be done in order to give you the time you need to recover and regenerate your cells.

How Does Your Vagus Nerve Deregulate Itself?

There is a fine balance between the sympathetic and parasympathetic nervous systems, and both work together to make sure you are able to survive in your environment. However, problems arise when your circumstances are such that your sympathetic nervous system remains activated for long periods of time because you are unable to remove or escape the stressors that are stimulating it. We are surrounded by relentless pressure and tension: We have jobs, families, financial strains, and mental imbalances that puts us in a constant cycle of stress—and therefore sympathetic activation. According to polyvagal theory, it's impossible for our bodies to maintain this state of sympathetic activation, and our nervous systems are always looking for a way to return to homeostasis. As long as we have stressors in our environment, it is likely the ventral vagal nerve will remain inactive and we won't be able to reach a state of ventral vagal social engagement.

Testing Your Vagus Nerve

Your vagus nerve is often the root of many imbalances, especially if you have a low vagal tone. The good news is that you can re-regulate this nerve to improve your physical, mental, and emotional health. In order to do this, however, you first have to learn when, and if, your vagus nerve is at fault—and this can be done by testing it. There are several tests that can be used to test the efficiency of the vagus nerve, all of which are done by stimulating or observing one or more of the functions that the vagus nerve is responsible for. These include the observation of the uvula, gag reflex, trapezius muscle, heart rate variability.

Mouth and Throat Observation

Your ventral vagal nerve is responsible for the muscles in the throat, one of which controls the uvula. The uvula is a little flap of skin that hangs at the back of the throat and secretes saliva so that your mouth stays hydrated and you're able to better digest your food. It also forms part of your soft palate, and is responsible for preventing food and liquids from moving into your nasal cavity when you swallow.

For this exercise, you'll need a partner or a mirror:

1. Open your mouth wide and shine a flashlight onto the uvula at the back of the throat.

2. If necessary, flatten your tongue with your fingers or a tongue depressor to get a better view of the uvula.

3. Say "ah" a few times, and watch the movement of the uvula as you do.

4. If the uvula moves symmetrically up and down as you make the sounds, it means you're in a state of social engagement. However, if it deviates to one side, it is a sign of ventral vagal nerve dysfunction.

In addition to the uvula, observing other parts of the soft palate can also be a good indicator of whether or not someone has a dysfunctional vagus nerve. The soft palate is connected to the pharyngeal branch of the ventral vagal nerve, and the test can be performed as follows:

1. Repeat steps one to three of the above test; instead of observing the uvula; however, watch the movement of the soft palate at the back of the throat.

2. If the soft palate moves up on one side but not the other, it might be indicative of a dysfunction.

The ventral branch of the vagus nerve is also responsible for our ability to swallow and our gag reflex. Another way to test the vagus nerve is through this reflex:

1. Use a cotton swab to tickle the back of the throat and stimulate the gag reflex.

2. This action should make you gag; if it doesn't, you might have a possible vagus nerve dysfunction.

Heart Rate Variability

The dorsal vagal nerve is what puts us into a state of dorsal vagal shutdown. At the same time, this branch of the vagus nerve is also what controls the muscles of the lungs and heart. Typically, we track our *heart rate*, which is the number of beats our hearts give per minute. *Heart rate variability*, on the other hand, is a measure of the changes in time between each heartbeat. It can only be measured using specialized devices, and it's a good indicator of the relationship between the sympathetic and parasympathetic nervous systems.

The more consistent the time intervals between heartbeats are, the more often your sympathetic nervous system is activated and the lower your heart rate variability will be. This means you are stressed more often, and you have a lower vagal tone. On the other hand, the more often your parasympathetic nervous system is activated, the higher your heart rate variability will be because the time intervals between successive heartbeats will be longer. This is indicative of a healthy nervous system and good vagal tone as it means you are more relaxed. Heart rate variability may change from day to day, depending on the physical and mental state of your body. For instance, if you are ill, your heart rate variability may be lower than usual; however, it will typically return to normal as soon as the pressure on your body decreases and your health improves.

Heart rate variability is measured in milliseconds. It's said that anything between 0 and 50 is considered unhealthily low, while a healthy heart variability is more than 100 milliseconds. Anything in between 50 and 100 milliseconds is considered a compromised nervous system. The calculations for heart rate variability are normally done automatically by the devices that measure it, but in short, it's determined by a VO2Max test that determines the intervals between heartbeats. Today, heart rate variability can be informally assessed with apps developed specifically for your smartphone.

In order to measure your own heart rate variability, you can do the following:

1. Using a heart rate monitor—such as an electrocardiogram, smart watch, or chest monitor—you can measure your heart rate variability.

2. Track your heart rate variability over a period of time, such as a month.

3. Note any changes: If it increases, it means your sympathetic nervous system isn't activated as much, and your vagal tone is improving. Your heart rate variability might change from day to day depending on your exact circumstances, but it's possible to get an average if you measure it for a few days or weeks.

Keep in mind that the most accurate way to measure heart rate variability is with electrocardiograms, which are typically used by medical professionals. That being said, while the popular devices available to the wider market are not as accurate, they can still be a relatively good indicator of the health of your nervous system.

Trapezius Squeeze

The trapezius muscle is located in the back, and it extends from the base of the neck to the middle of the back. Without this muscle, you wouldn't be able to move your head, neck, arms, or shoulders, and it's therefore responsible for a lot of motor function in the upper torso. The section of the trapezius muscle located in the shoulders can also be used to test the vagus nerve:

1. Locate the trapezius muscle in your shoulders, right between your neck and the tops of your shoulders.

2. Ask a partner to stand behind you and squeeze this muscle on the right and left-hand sides at the same time.

3. If your muscles are equally tight on both sides, it means you are in a state of social engagement; if not, it means you might have a nerve dysfunction.

Ventral Brake

The *ventral brake* is part of the ventral vagal system, and it's what keeps the heart rate from climbing too high. The strength of the ventral brake is important, and it only functions as long as the ventral pathways are active. You can strengthen your ventral brake by accessing your ventral vagal system more often—and this is what the exercises in Chapters 7, 8, and 9 aim to do. It can also be trained by moving up and down the polyvagal ladder—from the ventral vagal state to the dorsal vagal state and back again—through a process known as *pendulation*. Alternatively, you can also allow yourself to access the dorsal vagal system little bits at a time through a process known as *titration* in order to increase its tone and make it easier to return to a state of social engagement. The ease with which you are able to move between the different states is therefore indicative of the strength of your ventral brake, and by extension the vagus nerve.

Chapter 6:

Important Considerations

When Healing the Vagus Nerve

You are about to embark on a journey to heal your vagus nerve, and this journey will be unique to you. However, there are certain practices everyone can try to employ in order to make the way back to health a little easier. These include:

- Keeping a journal to track your progress.

- Committing yourself, and structuring your exercises in such a way that it's sustainable and manageable.

- Listening to your body—it will tell you everything you need to know!

- Staying aware so that you can do what is right for you.

- Staying in flow with yourself and your body to make your journey as efficient as successful as it can possibly be.

Tips and Tricks

Keeping a Journal

The vagus nerve has an influence on your physical and emotional health, which means you should remain aware of your mind and body in your journey of healing. One way to do this is by keeping a journal of how you're feeling physically and emotionally on a daily basis, and how these feelings may change over time. For instance, you can make daily notes on your sleeping and eating habits, how your muscles feel, what your mood is like, and if you have any difficulty concentrating or remembering. If you have any specific symptoms—such as muscle tension or digestive problems—it is also important that you focus on these. In addition, if there are any drastic changes in your health—for example, if your mood suddenly changes or you note shifts in your symptoms—you can also jot this down and see if you can establish what triggered it. Keeping track of your health and symptoms will help you to determine if there are any more subtle, long-term changes that can be attributed to your vagal tone, as well as how your daily exercises are influencing your symptoms.

Commitment and Structure

Practices work best when you commit to them and when you develop a routine and structure to make sure you stick to them. For instance, you can find dedicated times to practice every day, or you can commit to doing exercises for a set amount of time. You don't have to spend hours toning your vagus nerve—just a few minutes will make a discernible difference in your physical and mental health, as well as your ability to self-regulate. If scheduling practices are overwhelming or too stressful for you, you can allow yourself more flexibility, provided you continue to remain committed. Live in awareness and mindfulness, and use the feedback you get from your own body to decide when it's the right time for you to practice.

Listen to Your Body

Your body speaks, and it's your responsibility to listen! In addition to paying attention to your overall, long-term health, you should also be attentive to any changes in your body and mind while you do the practices. Try to keep track of your breathing, your heart rate, and the sensations you feel throughout your body. Do you feel tingling anywhere? Do you feel any pain, and if so, where do you feel it? Can you feel your energy flowing, and where do you feel it flowing to? Do you feel any blockages in your body, and where are they? Has any part of your body become more relaxed? Did anything shift in your digestive system? Were there any specific emotions or thoughts triggered by the practice? You can make mental notes of these, or you can write them down in your journal. Knowing how the different exercises affect you will also help you determine what works best for you and what you should rather avoid.

Do What Feels Right

Part of your healing journey is discovering what feels right so that you can begin to build a sustainable practice—but part of this means knowing what "right" feels like. Firstly, remember what the purpose of your practices are: Healing your vagus nerve is synonymous with releasing stress and trauma from the body so that you can shift yourself out of fight, flight, or freeze mode. This means the practices you do should feel good and rewarding, and that you should feel nourished in body and mind once you have completed them.

At the same time, also keep in mind that starting a new practice—and sticking to it—won't always be easy. You should learn to discern between the discomfort of trying to build healthy new habits and the type of pain that might mean the practices you're doing aren't working for your body. The most difficult choices in life are usually the choices that are the best and healthiest for us, but at the end of the day, you should still feel better when you're finished than how you did when you started. Anything that increases your stress or pain levels should be avoided at all costs—you don't want to worsen your trauma by not listening to your body.

Stay in Flow

Your body is a magical and complex system of billions of different parts, all of which have come together to create you as a physical, intellectual, and emotional being. Because of this complexity, what works for you one day might not work for you the next—and this is okay. Don't be too rigid, and give yourself the space and the grace to prioritize your wants, needs, comforts, and health. Listen to your body and do what feels good, and always remember there is no shame in stopping and starting again. An attitude of mindfulness and awareness will go a long way to staying in flow with yourself, and developing a sustainable practice that truly helps you to heal your body.

Chapter 7:

Three Minute Exercises to

Tone the Vagus Nerve

The vagus nerve is an important part of our body's communication system, and vagal dysfunction can have serious consequences for our physical, mental, and emotional health. The good news is that the vagus nerve can be toned to improve its response to stress, and thereby increase its efficiency in calming down the body in a healthy way. There are countless exercises that can relax and destress the body and mind, but some of the simplest include:

- eye movements

- breathwork

- SCM exercises

- spinal release exercises

- self-massage

- vocalization and throat stimulation

- cold exposure

Traditionally, the trauma stored in our vagus nerve would be addressed through talk therapy as a way to understand what caused it. The purpose of these exercises, however, is to address imbalances at a neurological level. They are simple to understand and perform, and best of all, they can be done in three minutes or less! This means they can be done daily and in almost any type of space—and all that's needed from you is the commitment to heal yourself.

The Importance of Commitment

Life is busy, and sometimes, even three minutes can seem like a lot. Don't let this get in your way—you owe it to yourself and your loved ones to stay healthy, happy, and productive. There's an assumption that the busier we are, the less time we can afford to spend on the things that benefit our health, such as exercises to tone our vagus nerves. However, consider this: A toned vagus nerve will result in better overall functioning, which can improve your productivity, save you time, and strengthen your relationships with loved ones. The irony of looking after yourself is that spending time on things that serve you will make your life easier in the long run, even if it requires some sacrifice now. Thankfully, these exercises are so short that it's not difficult to squeeze them into your daily schedule. Some of them can also be performed anywhere, and with minimal or no equipment—which means with the right knowledge and attitude, improved physical, mental, and emotional health is accessible to everyone.

The exercises outlined below are quick and easy. At the same time, you can't expect them to have any meaningful impact on your vagus nerve if you do them only once or twice. Like exercising anything else in your body, toning your vagus nerve takes patience and consistency, and most of all, commitment. Results won't come overnight, but if you stick with your practice long enough, they will come—guaranteed. If you commit yourself to doing them regularly, performing these exercises will soon become a daily habit... and once you begin reaping the benefits of these practices, it's a near-guarantee that you'll want to stick with them. Remember that a bucket is filled by a collection of little drops, and even the smallest of actions will amount to cumulative changes in the future.

Three Minute Exercises

Eye Movement

Eye movements are a very popular exercise, mostly because they are both easy and effective. They act as a "reset button" for the nervous system because the ventral vagal nerve is responsible for many of the functions that occur above the diaphragm, including the muscles of the eyes. Our eyes are closely associated with courage, as they are what scans the environment around us at all times. This means they also have a close link to our fight-or-flight response. The benefits of these exercises are that they help you to break tension patterns in your neck and shoulders. They can also shift your nervous system from a state of sympathetic activation to a calmer, more socially engaging neural circuit.

<u>Here is the "basic exercise" to tone your vagus nerve:</u>

1. First establish your "baseline" by turning your head to one side slowly without moving your body, and then turning it slowly to the other side. Sit up straight while doing this, and notice if there are any differences between the two sides. Is your neck tighter on one side than the other?

2. Next, lie down on your back with your knees bent or your legs straight, depending on what is more comfortable for you.

3. Interlace your fingers and place them behind your head; cradle your head in your fingers so that your thumbs rest on your neck just below your hairline.

4. Make sure your arms are relaxed and your elbows are wide.

5. Point your nose directly up to the sky.

6. Move your eyes to the right and up without moving your head. You can blink, but do not change the position of your eyes. It should be a comfortable position to hold, and you can use your hands to hold your head still.

7. Hold your eyes in place for 30 to 45 seconds, or until you feel the urge to sigh, yawn, or swallow—these actions indicate that you have reset your nervous system. When you are ready, bring your eyes back to the center.

8. Next, turn your gaze to the other side and repeat the process.

9. Once you are finished, sit up straight and try to turn your head from side to side again without moving your body, like you did in the beginning. Has it become easier than it was the first time? Do both sides feel the same this time around?

Variations to the "Basic Exercise"

1. As you become more used to the exercise, you can begin by doing it sitting upright, or even standing.

2. Place your hand on the side of your head and gently hold it there—this action should not cause any pain! Now tilt your eyes upward for 30 seconds. Repeat by tilting your head to the other shoulder and moving your eyes in the other direction. If you feel any strain or discomfort in your eyes, make the movement smaller— there is no need to push yourself too hard and a smaller

movement will have the same effect. Always remember to remain mindful of your body and to stay in flow with yourself. One of the key aspects of this journey is to listen to yourself—remember, the body doesn't lie.

Breathwork

Traditionally, breathwork—or breathing techniques—is known as *pranayama*. It is an ancient practice that has been around for thousands of years, and there is definite merit to it. There are many types of breathwork, all focusing on different outcomes or parts of the body. When it comes to the vagus nerve specifically, the purpose of using your breath is to engage your diaphragm, which is controlled to a large extent by your parasympathetic nervous system. This tones your vagus nerve and allows your body to slow down and relax. In addition to its physiological benefits, breathwork can also have a positive impact on your mind and emotions. Your brain is only able to focus on one thing at a time. If you are stressed, breathwork can take your attention away from the stressor and instead focus it on your body. The repetitive, rhythmic action of breathing therefore changes the mental space in which you are in, and allows your parasympathetic nervous system to take over. Breathing can also take your mind away from physical pain, and it's something you can easily do whenever you feel you need to activate your ventral vagal nerve.

Despite being a relaxation technique, breathwork can feel very uncomfortable, especially if you're not used to it. Additionally, it can also make you feel light-headed. Give yourself time to re-regulate your body after a breathwork session, and don't jump back into life too quickly. If you're new to the practice, take it slowly—if you feel you've had enough for one day, take a step back and return to it tomorrow: The most sustainable changes are made through small, consistent efforts.

Diaphragmatic Breathing

Diaphragmatic breathing—or belly breathing—is a type of breathwork that focuses on using the diaphragm. Your diaphragm is a muscle located between your abdomen and chest cavity, and it's responsible for helping you to breathe in and out. The first key to successful breathwork is to pay attention to where in the body you're sending your breath to. Another factor is the lengths of your inhales and exhales. Generally, people tend to believe that it's inhaling that relaxes your body. In reality, however, it's the exhale that is responsible for relaxing us.

Diaphragmatic breathing is one of the simplest breathwork exercises, and it can be done anywhere and at any time:

1. Sit or lie down comfortably and close your eyes.

2. Put one hand on your chest and the other on your stomach.

3. The key is to breathe with your abdomen and not your chest: Use your hands to regulate this by making sure that only the hand on your stomach moves when you breathe in and out.

4. Take a deep breath in through your nose for four counts, and feel your abdomen and rib cage expand.

5. Hold your breath on the inhale for two counts.

6. Exhale through your nose for six counts and feel your abdomen and rib cage contract. Make sure your mouth stays closed throughout the entire exercise.

7. Hold your breath on the exhale for two counts.

8. Repeat the exercise five to fifteen times, depending on how comfortable you are with breathwork.

Box Breath

Box breathing—or square breathing—is named as such because if you imagined the breathing pattern as a series of lines, it would form a box. It's helpful for relaxation because it focuses your attention on something other than your stressors, and it tricks your sympathetic nervous into calming down because it creates the impression of safety. Box breathing is incredibly simple, and can be done anywhere and at any time:

1. Sit or lie down in a comfortable place.

2. Inhale through your nose for four counts—remember to breathe all the way down to your navel, and not just into your chest. Imagine a line being drawn upward as you inhale to form the side of a "box."

3. Hold your breath on the inhale for four counts; again, imagine that same line drawing the top of the box.

4. Exhale through your nose for four counts and think of the line moving downward to form the other side of the box.

5. Hold your breath on the exhale for four counts, and imagine drawing the bottom of the box to end in the same place you started.

6. Repeat this exercise until you can start to feel changes in your body and your mood.

Hand Pressing Breath Exercise

This exercise uses breath to force your autonomic reflexes into action. It's simple and quick, yet very effective, and can be practiced by anyone, no matter how familiar you are with pranayamas. To do this exercise, make sure you are in a quiet place where you can focus on your breathing. Make yourself comfortable, and follow these steps:

1. Breathe in as deeply as you can.

2. Exhale slowly until your lungs are completely empty.

3. Hold your breath on the exhale and press your hands together.

4. Keep doing this for as long as you can; your autonomic reflexes will have been activated when you can no longer hold your breath, and your body is forced to take in large amounts of air.

5. Repeat this exercise as many times as you need in order to recenter yourself and calm your nervous system.

The Breath of Fire

The breath of fire is a popular method of breathing used in *kundalini yoga*, which is a practice dedicated to releasing energy and trauma that lies at the bottom of the spine or in the region of the navel. The purpose of this specific breathing technique is to detoxify your body and energize you so that you can rewire your nervous system. A further benefit of breath of fire is that it works some of your deepest core muscles, so the more you do it, the stronger you'll become physically. To access the energy that lies deep within your body, you can do the following:

1. Sit upright on the floor with your back as straight as possible. You can be in a cross-legged position, or if this is uncomfortable, you can elevate yourself slightly by sitting on a yoga block, a rolled-up blanket, or a cushion.

2. Start panting like a dog by giving short, sharp breaths.

3. Make sure you are breathing right down to your navel; you can do this by putting your one hand there to feel if

your stomach is expanding every time you inhale. Your inhale should be passive.

4. When you exhale, it should feel as if your navel is pulling to the back and toward your spine. The exhale must be active and forceful.

5. You should feel this exercise in your core, especially in your deeper abdominal muscles.

6. Try to increase your breathing rate—it may help to visualize a dog as you do it!

7. If breathing faster is difficult for you, slow down to a pace that works for you. It's always important to stay aware of your seating position and the depth of your breath—if you're starting out, it can be helpful to take it slowly at first. A slower breath with good form is still more effective than a fast breath with a compromised form.

8. Once you are sure that you are breathing all the way down to your navel, you can remove your hand and place your hands on your knees while at the same time bringing your thumb and ring finger together. You can also make your hands into fists and raise them into the air above your head.

9. Once you are ready to come out of the breath of fire, lower your chin to your chest, pull your navel to your spine, and pull your groin away from the floor in an upward direction; this will help you to lock your breath in place.

10. If your hands are in the air, you can push your thumbs together above your head while locking your breath.

The breath of fire is an incredibly powerful pranayama that can completely change your nervous system, and therefore your outlook on life. At the same time, it can also be dangerous for people who have respiratory infections, cardiac issues, or spinal injuries. In addition, pregnant women should also avoid performing this pranayama.

SCM Exercises

The *SCM* is the sternocleidomastoid muscle, which is located in the front of your neck. The SCM is the largest muscle in this region of your body, and it stretches from the top of your jaw to your collarbone. As a result, any tension here can lead to pain in your neck and head, as well as migraines and tension headaches. Your ventral vagal nerve is responsible for the motor functions of the SCM, and it can therefore be toned by releasing this muscle.

Variation I: Seated Upright

There are many different ways to release your SCM; when you have a few moments to yourself, try this easy seated stretch:

1. Sitting upright, bring your right ear to your right shoulder; it's important that you don't turn your head.

2. Shift your eyes as far to the right as you can without straining them.

3. Hold this position for five breaths, then repeat it by bringing your left ear to your left shoulder.

4. Next bring your right ear back to your right shoulder, but turn your gaze to the left.

5. Hold for another five breaths, then repeat it on the left-hand side.

Remember not to push or strain your muscles or your eyes— only do as much as you are comfortable with.

Variation II: Lying Down

If you have access to a place where you can lie down comfortably, you can use the following exercise to reset your SCM and activate your vagus nerve is by doing the following exercise:

1. Lie down on your stomach on a comfortable surface such as a carpet or a yoga mat.

2. Lift your upper body up by placing your elbows directly underneath your shoulders and your forearms parallel to each other in front of you.

3. While lifting your upper body — without straining yourself! — lift your head and turn it to the right as much as you can and look over your shoulder. Focus on the muscles in the side of your neck, and make sure you're using them to move your head in place.

4. Hold this position for 30 seconds, or until you feel a change in your body.

5. Release your head to the center, and repeat on the other side.

Releasing the Spine

The following exercise is a combination of the eye movements described above, and a lateral spinal movement. The benefit of this exercise is that it releases tension in your neck, shoulders, and back. It also tones the vagus nerve and stimulates the ventral vagal part of the parasympathetic nervous system:

1. Sit down in an upright position.

2. Put your left hand on the top of your head.

3. Place your right hand on the left side of your ribcage.

4. Using your left hand, gently pull your head down to your left shoulder.

5. At the same time, use your right hand to pull your rib cage to the right; imagine you are pulling your spine into a C-shape.

6. Turn your eyes up to the ceiling and hold them in place for a minimum of 30 seconds, or until you start noticing a change in your body.

7. Release your eyes back to look in front of your, and let go of your head and your rib cage.

8. Now, repeat this on the other side.

9. Make your movements as small as you need them to be; if you feel any pain, let go a little to a place where you feel comfortable again.

Self-Massage

Your vagus nerve is connected to a large number of muscles in your body, which means it can be reached through massage. A massage doesn't have to take up a lot of time or money, and best of all, if you know how, you can do it yourself! In addition, your vagus nerve is also connected to *fascia*, which is the thin layer of connective tissue that holds all of your organs, muscles, bones, vessels, and nerves in place. Fascia has both sensory and motor functions, but its most important role is to communicate events that happen inside the body to the brain. Because of this close relationship between fascia and the vagus nerve, it's possible to access the latter by physically massaging the first.

There is value in doing these exercises whenever you feel stressed, but there are even more benefits in doing them on a regular basis. Self-massage is not only a great way to build up your body's somatic memory so that it becomes easier to return to a place of calm, but it also increases your connection with yourself. For some of these exercises, you might need some equipment, such as massage balls or foam rollers. If you don't have these, don't stress—your fingers and hands can work just as well.

Fascia Facial Massage

One of the many functions controlled by the vagus nerve is the muscles in the face. These muscles often store a lot of tension, which can be released by massaging the right spots. This type of facial massage returns your body to a state of rest and relaxation, and improves your facial mobility so that you have more control over, and a greater diversity of, facial expressions. A facial massage requires you to focus on the following places:

1. The *TMJ* is a joint located at the point where your jaw is attached to your skull.

    a. Find this joint with your forefingers, then slide them forward to the place where you would ordinarily clench your teeth.

    b. Turn your forefingers inward with your palms facing you, and pull your cheeks back toward your TMJ and your ears in line with your teeth; start opening and closing your mouth slowly.

    c. Jut your jaw to the front and the back, as well as side to side to stimulate the muscles in your mouth while holding your cheeks in place.

    d. If you are using massaging balls, you can rotate them in this area; alternatively, if you're using your fingers, you can twist them in place.

2. The muscles that you use to scrunch your nose are located at the edges of the bottom of your nose. Place your fingers on these muscles so that they face toward the top of your nose.

     a.   Let your head hang down so that your fingers push the flesh next to your nose upward.

     b.   If you are using massage balls, lean your skull into them and gently twist them.

3.   The procerus muscle is located where the forehead meets the top of the nose—on your third eye—and it's one of the muscles you use to frown.

     a.   Place your thumb on your third eye with the nail facing downward, and gently twist it from side to side.

     b.   Alternatively, place one of the massage balls on this spot, and twist it slowly to massage and release the muscle.

4.   The muscles that line your temples can store a lot of tension, and it's important that they receive some attention, too.

     a.   Place your second and third fingers on your temples, next to your eyes, and twist them backwards and forwards.

     b.   Using your thumb and forefinger, you can also pinch the skin in this region to massage the temples.

     c.   If you're using massage balls, place them on your temples and twist them around.

5.   To massage your ears, place your fingers in the shells of your ears—not the tunnel—and move them around the different channels for as long as you feel necessary.

Myofascial Massage

The vagus nerve is connected to many parts of your body, and its ventral branch in particular forms part of the area around your collarbone, your chest and rib cage, and the part of your abdomen below your diaphragm. Each of these areas can be massaged individually to activate and re-regulate the vagus nerve and induce a sense of relaxation:

1. Your *supraclavicular zone* is the area around your neck and chest. To massage this zone, you'll need a coregeous ball:

   a. Put the ball against the side of your throat and face your head in the opposite direction.

   b. Gently twist it and roll it across the front of your throat to the other side.

   c. Move your head to the other side while moving the ball.

   d. Continue moving the ball back and forth; you can increase your pressure as you begin to warm up the tissue.

   e. Ideally, you should note a change in your neck and face, as well as in the quality of your voice.

2. The second important region for vagus nerve toning is the area around your ribcage and diaphragm, or your *thoracic zone*. Your vagus nerve is connected to both your lungs and diaphragm, and it can be accessed by moving the muscles in these areas using your breath.

   a. Lie down on your right side with the ball directly underneath your rib cage.

   b. Rest your right shoulder and arm on the ground, and place your head on top of your arm. Put your left hand on the side of your left rib cage.

   c. Take a deep breath; you should feel the muscles of your rib cage contracting with your left hand as your chest expands.

d. Exhale to let as much air out of your lungs as you can; feel your rib cage and chest contracting when you do this.

e. Repeat for eight to ten rounds on one side, or until you feel a noticeable change.

f. Repeat on the other side.

3. The *subdiaphragmatic zone* is below the diaphragm, around your gut and stomach. Many of the organs controlled by the vagus nerve are in this region, which is why focusing on this area is a good way to stimulate and tone the vagus nerve.

a. Lie face down with the ball underneath your stomach.

b. Rest your upper body on your elbows. Depending on the amount of pressure you want from the ball, you can either keep your torso raised, or you can rest your head on your forearms.

c. Take a deep breath in and contract your core muscles.

d. Release your core muscles as you exhale.

e. Repeat this as many times as you want; you can increase the pressure as you start to get used to the movement.

Vocalization and Throat Stimulation

Because your vagus nerve is connected to your vocal cords, you can access it through vocalization, such as humming and singing! Using your vocal cords activates the muscles in this region, which in turn stimulates and tones the vagus nerve. In addition, vocalization can also relax and soothe you because it regulates your breathing.

Humming and Chanting

Humming and chanting cause a lot of vibration in your body, especially in your ears, throat, and chest. This sensation stimulates and tones your vagus nerve, and helps your body to relax. Many of us may hum occasionally without even realizing it. However, if humming doesn't come to you naturally, try making the following sounds:

1. Take a deep inhale; keep your mouth closed as you slowly exhale to make a "m" sound. Continue making the sound for as long as you can. When you run out of breath, take another inhale and start again.

2. To make an "a" sound, take a deep breath in and open the back of your throat by imagining there's a ball there. Vocalize as you breathe out, and continue to focus on stretching the back of the inside of your throat while you do this.

3. Purse your lips together against the front of your teeth; first inhale, then make an "ou" sound as you exhale. Continue this for the entirety of your exhale, and repeat a few times.

4. Inhale once again, and use these three sounds to make a continuous "m-a-ou" sequence as you exhale. Move your mouth and jaw deliberately as you make these sounds, and focus on opening the back of your throat. You can turn this hum into a chant by continuously repeating the sound "om" until you feel your nervous system calm down.

This is a useful exercise, because the vagus nerve is not only activated by the vibration of the vocal cords, but also by the movement of the muscles in your jaw, throat, and lungs. Note any differences in your voice, as well as your breathing. You can do this exercise whenever and wherever you want, and you can repeat it as many times as you feel is necessary. It's quick, easy—and most of all, fun!

Singing

We haven't all been blessed with the ability to hold a tune, but that doesn't mean you can't sing! Singing stimulates the vagus nerve because it requires us to use our vocal cords, throat muscles, lungs, and diaphragm. Additionally, having fun to your favorite song can take your mind off your stress for a few minutes and instantly put you in a better mood. Find yourself some music you enjoy, turn up the volume, let go a little… and watch your nervous system transform itself.

Yawning

Yawning is a sign that our bodies and minds are tired, and that it's time for a break. Yawning is a reflex action that occurs when the vagus nerve is triggered, and that changes how blood flows and breath is taken up by the body. Studies also suggest that yawning is responsible for cooling down the brain when its temperature rises as a result of high metabolic rates. Because of this relationship between the vagus nerve and yawning, this reflex action can improve vagal tone.

Yawning often comes naturally, but by mimicking the actions you would normally take when you are about to yawn, you can induce yawning yourself. If your vagus nerve is in need of toning, bring relaxation to your body by trying the following:

1. Tilt your head back slightly and let your mouth hang open.

2. Contract the back of your throat while taking a deep breath in through your mouth.

3. When you feel the yawn coming on, allow it to happen: Let it stretch the muscles of your jaw and inflate your chest.

4. Feel the rush of breath as you exhale, and experience the sense of release that comes with it.

5. Repeat the exercise eight to ten times, or until your eyes start to tear up.

Gargling

Technically not a form of vocalization, however, gargling fluids also activates our vocal cords and the muscles at the back of our throats. As a result, it can have positive effects on the nervous system. If you've never gargled before, try the following:

1. Take a small to medium-sized sip of fluid, such as water. The fluid should be at a comfortable temperature.

2. Put your head back while simultaneously closing your throat so that you don't swallow the fluid.

3. Exhale while keeping your mouth open, and feel the bubbles in the back of your throat!

4. Try to gargle for 30 seconds to a minute without stopping.

5. You can repeat this twice a day in the morning and evening when you brush your teeth.

Laughing

Laughing requires the use of your vocal cords and diaphragm, both of which are closely associated with the vagus nerve. Activating these muscles can activate the parasympathetic nervous system and elevate you to a place of social engagement. In addition, the associations we have with laughter—joy, happiness, fun, and connection—further help to stimulate your ventral vagal circuit.

Laughter normally occurs organically, but it is possible to laugh intentionally. There are different types of laughing practices, and the secret is to find the one that works best for you. Laughing practice works best when it's done first thing in the morning, so that it can set the tone for your day. When laughing, always focus on relaxing your jaw and opening your mouth wider. This will influence whether the laughter comes from your abdomen—where it will activate your diaphragm and in turn stimulate your vagus nerve—or simply from your chest and throat.

Calcutta Laughter

1. Put your hands up with your palms facing forward.

2. Say "ho ho" while pushing your palms forward and away from you every time you make the sound.

3. Follow this by saying "ha ha" and pushing your palms downward to the floor.

4. Keep your knees slightly bent and sway your body gently while doing the practice.

5. You can speed it up or repeat it as many times as you need; you can also create pauses in the practice during which you inhale and exhale deeply.

Very Good, Very Good, Yay!

1. Say the words, "Very good, very good," while clapping your hands together every time you start with "very."

2. Follow this up with "yay," and put your hands up in the air triumphantly.

3. Do this with as much enthusiasm as you can— remember to have fun!

Gibberish Talk

1. Talk "gibberish" by saying sounds and words that are incoherent. Do it as fast as you can.

2. Add hand motions to your talking.

Laughing Sounds

1. Simply make laughing sounds—such as "ha ha ha" or "hee hee hee" while relaxing your jaw and keeping your diaphragm activated.

2. Remember, your body doesn't know the difference between real laughter and motions that simply mimic laughter—so fake it!

When laughing, your clothing is important: Try not to wear anything that can hinder movement in your abdominal region, such as tight pants or belts. Over time, you can build up your own practice of solo laughter to tone your vagus nerve and improve your overall mental and emotional health. The ideal is to laugh for 15 minutes a day—time that can be interspersed with breathing exercises.

Cold Exposure

Cold water is a great way to access the vagus nerve, and it can put you in a state of social engagement by making you feel calmer. Colder temperatures lower sympathetic activity in the body, and allows the parasympathetic nervous system to take charge. It also has anti-inflammatory benefits for our muscles and tissues, and bathing in cold or ice water is a popular practice with both athletes and ancient yogis. There are varying degrees to which you can submerge your body in cold water, but something as simple as splashing your face with cold water increases vagal tone and decreases heart rate. Other ways to harness the benefits of cold exposure include cold showers, ice baths, and cryotherapy.

Cold Showers

Wim Hof is famous for having developed a system—known as the *Wim Hof Method*—which aims to optimize the human body's natural abilities using elements in the natural environment. His method comprises different parts, one of which is using cold showers to increase resilience and reduce stress in order to live a higher-quality life.

1. Take a normal shower and end it with 15 seconds of freezing cold water.

2. Increase the time from 15 seconds to 30 seconds after a few days; continue doing this incrementally as you become more comfortable with cold showers.

3. Hof recommends two to three minutes of cold water a day to make the most of the practice; you can even take an entire shower using just cold water.

If you don't want to commit your entire body to a cold shower, you can still get the benefits of cold exposure by immersing your face in cold water:

1. Pour two inches of cold water in a bucket or sink; the water should be as cold as possible, preferably 10-12°C.

2. Put your face in the water; make sure that your eyes, forehead, and at least two thirds of your cheeks are underwater.

3. Hold your face there for as long as your breath lasts, and come up for air when necessary.

4. Note any changes in your body: What is happening to your breathing and heart rate? Are there any changes in your digestive system? Do your muscles feel more relaxed?

5. Repeat the exercise as many times as you want, or until you start to notice changes in your body.

Cryotherapy

Cold therapy—or *cryotherapy*—is a practice that uses extreme cold to reduce blood flow to a certain region of the body. It can be localized or applied to the entire body, depending on the area you aim to address, and it can be done using ice packs, cold air, coolant sprays, ice massage, ice baths, or through probes medically inserted into the body. When it comes to nerve disorders—and in particular vagus nerve dysfunction—cryotherapy is useful because the cold makes the organs that are connected to the vagus nerve, such as the chest and digestive muscles, send distress signals to the brain. This "resets" the body by activating the vagus nerve and turning down the body's stress response. In addition to reducing stress levels, cryotherapy is also good for treating inflammation and helping to regulate mood and attention.

Cryotherapy can be done in many ways, but there's a simple way to use the cold to activate the vagus nerve at home:

1. Find a bowl that is large enough for you to put your face in.

2. Fill the bowl with ice and water to whatever ration suits you.

3. Set a timer for between 15 and 30 seconds; take a deep breath in and put your face in the water.

4. Keep your face underwater until the timer goes off.

5. Note the changes in your body—you should find that your heart rate has decreased, your ability to focus has increased, and your stress levels are lower.

Ice Baths

1. Your body will be shocked, but focus on trying to slow your breath and staying calm.

2. Time yourself, and stay in the bath for as long as you can. Try to stay in the water for a little longer every time you take an ice bath—but don't push yourself too hard!

3. Ice baths can be taken for six to eight minutes at a time up to four times a week, depending on how new you are to the practice.

Ice baths are a useful way to stimulate the vagus nerve, but if you suffer from high blood pressure or pre-existing cardiovascular conditions, cold exposure can increase your risk for strokes and cardiac arrest. A further risk with cold exposure is hypothermia, which occurs when your body loses too much body heat without being able to restore it; this is especially true if you remain submerged in the ice bath for too long. Anyone with type 1 or 2 diabetes should also be careful when exposing themselves to cold temperatures, because these conditions are associated with a reduced ability to maintain core temperatures during extreme temperature changes.

Chapter 8:

Long(er) Exercises to Stimulate and Strengthen the Vagus Nerve

Toning your vagus nerve using the quick and easy exercises described in Chapter 7 can be very helpful in the long-term. That being said, some people may be looking for a little more—which is what this chapter is all about. The exercises below can be as long or as short as you want them to be, and they include:

- meditation

- yoga

- *tai chi*

- *qigong*

- facial muscle release

As always, it's important to listen to your body—stay aware and mindful, and only do as much as you're comfortable with.

Vagus Nerve Exercises

Meditation

In its broadest sense, the purpose of meditation is to train your attention and focus so that you can restore a sense of calm and balance to your life. Meditation has been around for thousands of years—especially in Asia—and it forms a central part of many religions. The mental and emotional benefits of meditations are endless: It can teach you to live in the present so that you have a fuller experience of life, and it can increase your compassion, joy, and ability to connect. Scientifically speaking, meditation also has a positive effect on the physical body—specifically, the vagus nerve. There are many different types of meditation and each serves its own unique purpose. In general, meditation places awareness on breathing and heart rate. As a result, this practice helps to tone the vagus nerve because it is so closely associated with these two organs.

Some of the most popular meditative techniques used to tone the vagus nerve include somatic meditation, mindfulness meditation, and mantra meditation.

Somatic Meditation

The word *somatic* is related to our sensory experience, so the purpose of somatic meditation is therefore to turn your focus to any internal sensations you may be experiencing. These could include the rhythmic beating of your heart, the sound of your pulse in your ears, the weight of your body resting on the earth, and tingling in your fingers and toes. In addition, the aim is also to pay attention to the sounds, smells, temperature, and textures around you. Somatic meditation is all about remaining in the present moment, and directing your attention toward your body, rather than your thoughts.

Trauma disconnects us from our external environment, and it tends to distract or remove us from the present moment. By turning your attention toward the sensation in and around your body, you can begin to release the stress and tension you're storing inside you. Regarding your vagus nerve, somatic meditation activates neuroception by connecting yourself to your senses. This creates a sense of safety which relaxes your body and releases the stress that you store inside you.

1. Find yourself in a comfortable seated position in a peaceful environment.

2. If you're wearing glasses, remove them. Next, focus on the sights around you: Keep your eyes open and look at your environment. Take note of the things that draw your attention most—what are their colors, textures, and shapes? Try not to think about these objects; instead, simply let your eyes wander around and rest on whatever they want to, for as long as you feel necessary.

3. Wiggle your toes and fingers, and allow your body to feel the textures around you. What does the surface underneath feel like? What is the temperature on your skin? What do your clothes feel like on your body?

4. Again, pay attention to the feelings and textures that catch your attention, and linger on them until you feel it's time to move on.

5. Turn your focus to the inside of your body, and notice any sensations you may be feeling. Can you feel or hear your heartbeat? Does it feel as if there's a tightness in your chest, or any movement in your stomach? Is your breath fast or slow, or deep or shallow, and does this affect the movement of your ribcage and the skin on your back? Do you have tightness or pain in your body,

or do you feel more relaxed in some places than others? Is there any tingling in your body?

6. Try to create a mindful connection between your external environment and your inner sensations. Think about how you reacted when you turned inward: Did you forget about the textures and sights around you, or were you able to incorporate them with the sensations in your body?

7. Once you have felt the inside of your body, revisit the sights and textures that attracted you the most before.

8. Keeping your eyes open, continue to focus on your external environment while once again turning inward. See if you can remain mindful of all these experiences at the same time. It might help to move your body in subtle ways, like wiggling your toes and fingers, or slowly swaying from side to side.

9. Don't force your attention in any direction—remember, the aim is simply to observe.

10. It's possible for the sensations in your body to shift while you're observing them. Try to notice these changes as they happen. If you feel any negative sensations, such as pain, acknowledge it for a moment without lingering on it.

11. Start to focus on the sounds around you, especially those that are the quietest. Keep your eyes open while you tune into the most subtle sound you can hear, and try to maintain your connection to your internal body while you do this.

12. Shift your attention to the loudest sound you can hear, and let it absorb you for a moment.

13. Think of the direction from which these sounds—the softest and the loudest—are coming. Are they coming from the same side of your body, or from opposite

sides? Try to use your ears to focus on sounds coming from the left and right sides at the same time. What is your experience of doing this? Is it difficult to use both your sides at the same time? Do you struggle to shift from the left to the right, or vice versa? Is one side more dominant than the other?

14. Notice any movement that might be happening in your body, such as turning your head, stretching your neck or back, or shifting around in your seat.

15. If your head wants to move in a specific direction, let it slowly go where it wants to.

16. Allow your body to move how it wants: Stretch your arms, move your hands and feet, shift your torso forwards and backwards… if you don't feel the urge to move, don't—just let your body do what it wants to.

17. Slow down your movement and return your attention to whatever attracts it the most. Has your focus shifted? Is your experience of the sights, sounds, and feelings around you different than it was before?

18. Once again, turn inward, and notice if the sensations you felt before have changed.

19. Continue this exercise for as long as you want to.

Because you are trying to cultivate a connection with what is around you, it's helpful to keep your eyes open as much as you can. Also, remember not to force your attention in any specific direction, or to think about what you're experiencing. Stay present and gentle, and shift your focus around slowly so that you can receive as much sensory information as you can. The key is awareness and mindfulness, and to allow your body and mind to move and linger in a way that feels natural and organic to you.

Mindfulness Meditation

The art of mindfulness is all about staying in the present moment. This includes letting go of past sadness or future worries. Mindfulness meditation is a combination of the art of staying present and the training and focus required by meditative practices. Its purpose is to slow down your thoughts and situate you in the present so that you can come to a calmer place. This shift in focus, combined with the stimulation of your heart and lungs through mindful breathing, activates the ventral vagal nerve and puts you in a state of social engagement. This practice also aims to help you accept your thoughts and feelings without being harsh on, or judgmental of, yourself. Mindfulness meditation is therefore a wonderful way to stop racing thoughts and reconnect with your body and your environment.

There are many variations of mindfulness meditation, but the simplest practices don't require any props, aside from a comfortable place to sit. In addition, you can meditate for as long as you need—three minutes of breath and focus is enough to improve your health. A session of mindfulness meditation might follow these steps:

1. Sit down in a comfortable position; make sure your spine is straight and your arms and shoulders are relaxed.

2. Close your eyes and focus all of your attention on the present moment.

3. Begin by focusing on your breath: Feel your body move as you inhale, and hear the rush of air as you exhale. Breathe naturally, and continue to let yourself be absorbed by the organic flow of your breathing.

4. Bring your attention to the top of your head: What does your scalp feel like? Is there any tingling, or vibrations? Are there no sensations in this part of your body?

5. Move your attention to your forehead, then your eyes, nose, jaw, cheeks, mouth, and chin. Linger in each area for a while, and try to absorb all the sensations you feel. Don't make any judgments—simply embrace and accept the present moment for what it is.

6. Next, move to your torso: Your neck, your collar bone, your left shoulder, arm, elbow, wrist, palm, fingers... scan your body in this way as you slowly shift your attention from one place to the next, ending with the tips of your toes. Linger for as long as you want, and move on when you are ready.

7. Don't ignore any thoughts that come up—imagine you're sitting on a riverbank, and your thoughts are floating past you... acknowledge them, and then let them go.

8. If you find your mind wandering, simply bring it back to the present and continue with your body scan.

Mantra Meditation

Mantra meditation is a type of meditation practice that uses repetitive mantras as a way to focus attention and energy. It's particularly helpful if you have difficulty concentrating because focusing on a mantra can reduce wandering thoughts, and it can even help you improve other meditation practices. In addition, it's also a simple way to find a natural breathing rhythm. Mantra meditation has similar benefits to other styles of meditation, including relaxation and calm, a more positive lease on life, less stress, and increased self-awareness. In addition, it has advantages for your health, as it relaxes your nervous system and allows your body to enter a ventral vagal state of rest and digest.

The choice of mantra is entirely up to you. Some people prefer chanting a single word—such as "peace"—as a way to reaffirm what the aim of their meditation is. Others choose affirmations—such as "I am strong," or "I am compassionate"—as their mantras. You can even use a single syllable—"om," or "aum"—as part of your meditation practice. Ideally, your mantra should reflect your intentions, as repeating this over and over again will continually guide your attention in that direction.

A simple mantra meditation will unfold in the following way:

1. Find a comfortable seat.

2. Choose a mantra—remember to keep the intention of your practice in mind.

3. Decide how long you want your meditation to last, and set a timer. Alternatively, if you have no restrictions on your time, you can continue meditating for as long as it feels necessary.

4. Begin your meditation with a few deep breaths through your nose; try to find a natural breathing rhythm, and focus on the sensation of your breath moving in and out through your body.

5. Start chanting your mantra, either out loud or silently.

6. Continue the meditation, and notice how your chant and your breath begins to sync up.

7. Whenever your thoughts wander, acknowledge them and let them go; gently return your attention to your mantra.

8. Take a few moments at the end of your meditation to turn inward and assess your body and mind. How do

you feel? What is your mood? What has meditation done to your heart rate and breath? Do you feel more positive and optimistic? Do you feel more relaxed? Use the answers to these questions to track your progress as you continue to build on your practice.

Yoga

Yoga is a wonderful way to tone your vagus nerve, because the combination of breath and movement becomes a moving meditation. Personally, I consider yoga to be a practice that strengthens the body and the mind. Because it can be practiced in a community of like-minded people, it also encourages co-regulation. Additionally, yoga supports self-awareness, self-compassion, and mindfulness practices.

In Western traditions, the focus of yoga is often on its purely physical aspects; however, if you dig deeper into the practice, you'll find there's much more to it than that. In Sanskrit, *yoga* means "yoke," or "wholeness." When you consider the impact many of these poses have on your physical and mental health, that's exactly what yoga is: A coming together of the different parts of the body so that they can once again function in harmony and balance.

There are many different yoga poses, and some of them are more advanced than others. Fortunately, there are very simple yoga poses that can be performed by anyone—even beginners—and you don't have to be a seasoned yogi to heal your vagus nerve using this ancient practice. There are also many different ways in which these poses can be put together; for instance, they can be performed in isolation, or they can be put together in a flow to form one continuous sequence of movement.

There is no prescription for how long each pose should be held. The secret to using this practice to successfully heal your vagus nerve is to listen to your body, and to only do as much as you're able to. Never, ever push yourself beyond your own limits, because injury won't serve you in any way. Also keep in mind that your body changes from day to day, so you might be capable of doing more on one day than you will on another. "Deeper doesn't always mean better," and the key to healing yourself is to respect your own limits.

Poses and Postures

One of the most important aspects of yoga is movement. There are hundreds of yoga poses ranging from very simple to extremely advanced; however, even a newcomer to the practice can tone their vagus nerve and get the countless health benefits of yoga without risking injury or putting themselves in an uncomfortable position. Some of the most popular yoga poses—and the most effective for healing vagal dysfunction—include:

- cat cow
- happy baby pose
- warrior I
- warrior II
- cobra pose
- sphinx pose
- upward-facing dog
- camel pose
- reverse table pose
- bridge pose

- seated side bends

- seated forward fold

- seated twists

- child's pose

- waterfall

- bow pose

- seated backbend

- downward-facing dog

Yoga classes and flows are greatly dependent on individual needs, but most traditional yoga classes will follow the same sequence:

1. Begin in a seated position on your mat; take time to quiet your mind and set an intention for your practice. This portion of the class can even involve a quick meditation, if your body and mind call for it.

2. Start your movement with a few stretching poses to warm up your body; these can include child's pose, cat cow, seated side bends, hero pose, and stretches for your wrists in dynamic table top pose.

3. Once your body is ready, begin the chosen yoga flow. Some examples include sun salutations or moon salutations, but it doesn't have to be—listen to your body, and give it what it needs!

4. End your yoga flow in corpse pose, or *savasana*: This is performed by lying flat on your back with your legs outstretched, and your arms relaxed to the sides of your body. Your savasana can last as long as you need it to, and it's best not to force yourself out of it too soon.

5. Slowly come back to your body once your savasana is finished; return to a seated position on your mat.

6. Sit quietly for one minute before you resume your day.

There are thousands of different yoga flows and sequences, all of which serve different purposes. The following sequence is useful for stimulating the vagus nerve:

1. Begin in mountain pose, with your arms to the side and your feet grounded in the earth.

2. On an inhale, raise your arms to the sky, then exhale and fold forward over your legs so that your fingertips face the floor.

3. Place your palms on the ground in front of you, and step back into downward-facing dog.

4. From downward-facing dog, slide forward into plank. Press out of your shoulders and be careful not to sag your back and stomach.

5. Step your right foot between your hands. Rise into a high lunge with your arms in the air above your head. Make sure your knee is stacked directly above your ankle, and try to keep your shoulders relaxed and away from your ears.

6. Place your left hand on the floor beside your right foot, and raise your right hand in the air to open your chest.

7. Return to your high lunge.

8. Place your hands on the floor on either side of your foot and step your right foot back to meet your left; return to plank position.

9. On an exhale, return to downward-facing dog.

10. Repeat the sequence on the other side by once again moving into plank and stepping your left foot in between your hands. End in downward-facing dog.

11. Slowly, walk your feet forward to meet your hands; find yourself in a forward fold.

12. Come to the ground in a seated position with your legs crossed.

13. Place your right hand on your left knee, and your left hand behind you on the floor. On an exhale, twist your torso to the left, and stay here for a few breaths. Work with your breath: lengthen when you inhale, and twist deeper when you exhale. Return to the center.

14. Reverse the cross of your legs, and repeat the twist on the other side.

15. Lie down on your back with your knees bent in front of you and your hands facing down to the sides of your body; your feet should be flat on the floor and hip's width apart.

16. Move into bridge pose by raising your hips in the air, vertebrate by vertebrate. Your head, neck, and shoulders should remain on the ground. Try to push into the soles of your feet and the palms of your hands to raise yourself a little higher.

17. Slowly roll down, starting from the top of your body all the way down to the small of your back. You should once again be lying flat on your back.

18. Straighten your legs out in front of you, and place your hands facing upwards to the side for savasana. Relax your body and feel yourself melt into the ground. Stay here for a few minutes.

19. Return to your body slowly by wiggling your toes and fingers. Keeping your eyes closed, roll to the side and push yourself back up into a seated position.

20. Remain seated for one minute and feel the changes in your body.

Remember to listen to your body: Discomfort is sometimes a natural part of movement, but pain shouldn't be. If any of these poses causes you agony, let it go, and try something else. The wonderful thing about yoga is there's something for everyone!

Ujjayi Breathing

In addition to movement, another essential part of yoga is breathwork. *Ujjayi breathing*—also called ocean breath—is a soft, whispering form of breathing that mimics the sound of the ocean. It is one of the most common forms of yogic breathwork, and its aim is to focus your mind on your breath in order to calm and relax yourself. In addition, the distinct sound of this type of breathing also helps you to connect your body to the poses as you move through a yoga flow.

Ujjayi breathing is important for vagus nerve toning because it affects the breath, heart rate, and mind simultaneously. It can be performed in conjunction with a yoga flow, or on its own. To get started with *ujjayi* breathing, try the following:

1. Inhale through your nose, keeping your mouth closed.

2. Exhale through your nose, keeping your mouth closed.

3. As you exhale, constrict your throat so that your breath makes a rushing sound.

4. Breathe all the way into your abdomen—you can even place your hands on your stomach or rib cage to feel your body expand and contract as you inhale and exhale.

5. Your inhalations and exhalations should last the same amount of time, depending on what you find most comfortable.

Tai Chi

Many people describe *Tai chi* as "meditation in motion" because of its combination of movement, breath, and mindfulness. It's a low-impact and slow-paced form of exercise consisting of a series of poses that are all done in a continuous flow. The aim of *Tai chi* is to focus your attention on your breath and the sensation in your body. Although it is a form of exercise, *Tai chi* is practiced with relaxed muscles; this is why it can be done by most people, regardless of their physical abilities. Even so, *Tai chi* improves muscle strength, balance, flexibility, and aerobic fitness. In addition, it is also a great way to relax the nervous system and tone the vagus nerve.

Tai chi originated in ancient China as a martial art, but it has become a popular form of exercise in the West because of the health benefits derived from the mind-body connection the practice aims to cultivate. *Tai chi* is especially helpful in lowering blood pressure and reducing inflammation, both of which are common problems for someone with vagal nerve dysfunction. In addition, it can also be used as a form of preventative medicine to avoid health problems in the future.

Tai chi flows differ vastly, and should ideally be guided by professional practitioners. That being said, there are a few main principles that most flows take into account:

- Movements should be slow, smooth, and controlled; when moving, imagine you're pushing against a very light resistance, such as someone moving through water.

- The form and structure of your body is very important: Your posture should remain upright and aligned, and you should pay attention to how and where the weight in your body is transferred.

- Remember to keep your limbs slightly bent and your joints loose; don't lock out your knees or elbows, but also continue to make sure that your movements continue to be deliberate and strong.

- The purpose of *Tai chi* is to work on both the body and the mind, so aim to cultivate mental quietness by staying mindful and present.

QiGong

QiGong is a combination of meditation, movement, and controlled breathing used to heal the body, mind, and spirit. The word can roughly be translated to mean "the master of one's energy," and is an ancient Chinese practice aimed to use the energy of nature within one's body. Within the theory of *QiGong*, it's believed imbalances and health problems result from a blockage in the energy pathways within our bodies; the purpose of the practice is to release these blockages and promote better energy flow. *QiGong* can also be divided into two categories: *Active QiGong* involves movement and breathwork aimed to increase energy, and *passive QiGong* focuses on stillness and meditation to calm the body down.

While *QiGong* is an ancient practice with spiritual roots, it has great benefits for the vagus nerve. It incorporates movement, meditation, and breathing, all of which are cited as ways in which vagal tone can be improved. It stimulates the connective tissue, diaphragm, heart, and lungs, introduces slow, gentle movement into the body, and brings the mind to a place of mindfulness and rest. All of this helps to increase blood circulation, lower blood pressure, release feel-good hormones, and relax the nervous system. There are many ways in which *QiGong* can be practiced, but the following movements are helpful for toning the vagus nerve:

1. Begin by shaking out your entire body—including your hands, arms, feet, and legs—to release anxiety and tension.

2. Place your palms together in front of the space of your heart, and rotate them in opposite directions.

3. Placing your hands in a prayer position, push them to the right while looking to the left, and repeat this on the other side; keep doing this as a smooth—but gentle—continuous movement. This will help to release your neck and improve your vagal tone.

4. Remember to connect with people, nature, and yourself as often as possible—healthy vagal tone begins when you feel safe and secure!

Facial Muscle Release

The vagus nerve can be stimulated through the face—which means facial massages and therapies are the perfect way to relax! In addition, they improve muscle tone in the face, increase blood flow, and invigorate the skin. There are many different face therapies available, and many of them are simple and quick enough that they can be done at home with minimal—or no—equipment and a little bit of research.

Gua Sha Tool

Gua sha is a practice that uses a flat jade pebble used to lightly scrape the skin of the face. Also known as *jade scraping*, it's an ancient Chinese healing practice that was originally used as a body treatment. One of the biggest benefits of *Gua Sha* is that it facilitates lymphatic drainage, which helps to reduce bloating. It also stimulates blood circulation in the face, helps the skin to produce collagen, and decreases inflammation in this region. *Gua Sha* has many advantages in terms of physical appearance, because it reduces puffiness and darkness, and it "chisels" the face by improving the tone of the facial muscles.

The vagus nerve can be activated through facial massage, which means regular *Gua Sha* treatments can go a long way to heal vagal dysfunction. At the same time, it can also be done by yourself at home, provided you have the right tool for the job:

1. Apply a small amount of facial oil to your face.

2. Using your gua sha tool, gently stroke the skin of your face in the direction of lymphatic flow.

3. You can combine short and long strokes, depending on what the specific area of your face requires; if it is uncomfortable or painful, it means you're pressing too hard.

4. Extend your strokes to include your neck and the upper part of your chest.

5. Your skin type will determine how often you should *Gua Sha*; however, it is typically recommended you do it once a week.

Avoid *Gua Sha* if you have sunburn or rashes. In addition, remember that there is no one-size-fits-all approach to *Gua Sha*, so remember to evaluate its effects on your body, and use these observations to establish a practice that works for you!

Facial Exercises and Face Yoga

Yoga, yoga everywhere… even for your face! *Face yoga* is the practice of massaging your face to stimulate the muscles and skin. This can help to firm and tone the face, and to reduce any dark circles. In addition, face yoga influences the lymphatic system, which means it helps with drainage and can reduce puffiness. Most importantly, face yoga is an effective way to tone the ventral vagal nerve and bring the body and mind to a state of rest and relaxation. Furthermore, it has an effect on your facial expressions, and can even help you reduce the number of times you activate the muscles used to express negative feelings, such as worry and anger. Face yoga can also be extended to include the neck and shoulders, and in addition to its many physiological benefits, this practice can also boost confidence and generate positivity. Some popular and effective poses include:

- lion pose

- puppet face

- baby bird

- big smile

- buddha face

Face yoga is also closely associated with *acupressure*, which is the use of pressure on targeted places in the body. Acupressure is typically performed using the fingers, palms, elbows, or other tools, depending on the specific pressure point that is being targeted. In addition to this practice, it is also recommended that face yoga be combined with other holistic activities such as good sleep hygiene and a healthy and balanced diet. Some of these activities are described in Chapter 9.

Chapter 9:

Additional Practices

Toning your vagus nerve is important to live a healthier and more stress-free life, but the healing journey doesn't stop there. If we want to truly live the healthiest lives we possibly can, we have to take into account everything we do on a daily basis. This includes:

- eating habits
- journaling and therapy
- our work-life balance and time management
- movement and exercise
- rest, relaxation, and sleep
- self-talk
- emotional and mental expression
- sexual release
- social engagements

No life can be lived flawlessly, and we all have habits we'd like to change. It's impossible to do everything right all the time, but living a healthy life is not about doing it perfectly—it's about continuing to try.

Living a Healthy Life

Healthy Eating Habits

Your mind is hosted by your body, which is in turn fueled by food; this means that your eating habits have an impact not only on your physical health, but also your mental and emotional wellbeing. Healthy eating habits differ from person to person, and each individual has their own unique nutritional needs. A few basic ideas include:

- Eating enough fruit and vegetables to nourish your body with the fiber, vitamins, and minerals it needs.

- Avoiding processed foods and excessive amounts of saturated and trans fats.

- Cutting back on sugar and artificial sweeteners.

- Avoiding refined carbohydrates.

- Reducing your meat intake, especially meats that contain harmful substances, especially red meat, charred meat, and processed meat.

- Limiting your alcohol intake and cigarette consumption, and avoiding any other chemical substances and drugs.

Journaling and Therapy

The purpose of journaling is to verbalize and express your thoughts, feelings, and ideas in a way and a place that feels comfortable to you. There are different types of journaling, such as reflective journaling, travel journaling, gratitude journaling, or stream of consciousness journaling. Journaling doesn't have to take up a lot of time, nor does it have to be very complex. All you need is some paper, a pen or pencil to write with, and a few minutes to yourself in a quiet place. If you struggle to get started, there are many sources that can help you to build a regular journaling practice.

Like journaling, therapy is also centered around expressing the thoughts and feelings that are causing imbalances in your life. In contrast to journaling, it also includes advice from a registered professional. Negative things happen to all of us, every day, and sometimes it's impossible for us to cope with these alone. There's no shame in asking for help—all it means is you care enough to maintain or improve your mental and emotional health.

Work-Life Balance and Time Management

Work is important, but so is taking a break from it. A *work-life balance* refers to the way you divide your time and focus between everything that requires it. This includes jobs, hobbies, friends, family, and time for reflection and self-care—all of which is necessary for physical and mental wellbeing. It's difficult to maintain a healthy work-life balance, especially given how busy our lives have become. However, with efficient time management strategies, you can create a sustainable schedule for yourself that gives you enough time to do the things that need to be done, while also allowing you to take a break from stressful activities by doing the things that stimulate and energize you.

Light Movement and Exercise

It's believed we need at least 30 minutes of exercise a day, even if it's only light movement. Exercise has countless benefits: It helps us to destress, it aids in digestion and circulation, it improves muscle strength, flexibility, and cardiovascular fitness, and it releases endorphins and hormones that help us to feel good about ourselves and our lives. It also energizes us and gives us an opportunity to learn new skills and test our abilities in new and unexpected ways. Exercise doesn't have to be a chore—there is something out there for everyone, and if you can find something you truly enjoy, regular exercise will stop feeling like a burden and instead turn into a privilege

Rest, Relaxation, and Sleep

We have all, at times, given up sleep for things that seemed more urgent. However, not getting enough rest is one of the biggest mistakes we can make. Our bodies and minds need time to regenerate and recover, and if they're forced to work constantly without any breaks, they stop functioning efficiently. It can be difficult to go to sleep knowing you have looming deadlines, but the reality is if you don't rest, your productivity and cognitive functioning can decrease to such an extent that you lose even more time than you would've spent sleeping. No matter how busy life gets, it's important that we give our bodies what they need—and that includes sufficient rest.

Self-Talk

Most of us would never say mean and degrading things to others, so why do we say them to ourselves? When you repeat something to yourself over and over again, the plasticity of your brain rewires itself so that over time, you become what you told yourself. Self-talk has an immense influence on how we view ourselves, and in turn, how we behave. If we constantly demean ourselves, we will come to believe it, and our ability to achieve will reflect it. On the other hand, if you have a good, positive relationship with yourself and you make a point of regularly uplifting yourself with affirmations and mantras, this too, will show up in your everyday life.

Feeling Your Feelings

Your feelings are a way for your mind to process events that are happening around you—so allow yourself to feel them! There is no weakness in anger, disappointment, or sadness; we all have things we need to process, and the only way to get over something is to move through it. That being said, wallowing in your feelings and using them as an excuse to hurt others or avoid life isn't healthy either, but that doesn't mean they should be suppressed. When we stop ourselves from feeling something, the feeling doesn't go away—it remains in our subconscious where it can cause physical, mental, and emotional pain. If you can find the courage to face up to your emotions, you will also find yourself living a healthier and more fulfilling life.

Sexual Release

Sex and masturbation are one of the most important yet least-talked-about aspects of health and wellbeing. It's a normal part of human physiology, and it has countless health benefits. For instance, regular sexual release can reduce pain, improve heart health, boost immunity, deepen connections with others, increase focus and memory, and regulate mood and emotions. Sexual intercourse and orgasms also physiologically stimulate the vagus nerve and increase the secretion of oxytocin. This hormone forms a vital part of our stress response, and it helps the body feel relaxed and sleepy. There are many ways to practice sex safely, and it doesn't always require a partner—so make the time to give your body what it needs!

Social Engagements

Human beings are social creatures, and whether we like it or not, we can't live without social interaction. Healthy and productive engagements with others encourages co-regulation, which helps us to feel safe and connected to other people. These feelings also pave the way for a ventral vagal state, and can improve our physical, mental, and emotional health. It also allows us to learn from others and increase our own knowledge-base. This also gives us an opportunity to express ourselves, our thoughts, and our ideas to someone who can respond to what we say. Social interactions don't have to be harrowing; the important thing is that you choose the people around you wisely, and that you spend time doing things you love in an environment that makes you feel safe and secure.

Conclusion

Our bodies are magical: We are made up of trillions of cells that come together in a unique way to allow us to think, feel, express, and move. Unfortunately, our bodies are not always in harmony, and this can cause us to suffer physical, mental, and emotional discomfort and pain. At the same time, these symptoms are signs from our bodies that something is wrong, and that it's time for us to change something we've been doing, or to implement something new in our lives. It's important to learn to listen to your body, because it will tell you everything you need to know. If you pay attention to how you feel—physically and emotionally—you can get to know yourself better over time. You will learn to know when you need rest, when you need to be active, and when you need to express how you feel so that you can begin to self-regulate and address any imbalances you might be suffering from.

The vagus nerve is an essential part of our physiology, and it influences a vast number of functions in the human body. Vagal dysfunction can give rise to a variety of physiological and psychological symptoms and result in the imbalances many of us suffer from. In order to know if it is indeed your vagus nerve that is causing your distress, it should be tested. This can be done using both simple or more complex methods.

Getting to know the source of your imbalances is only one part of the journey. The other—and most important—is to begin to incorporate practices that can help you heal your vagus nerve and address your physical and psychological imbalances. Establishing a new routine is not always easy, but the simple and effective ways to re-regulate your vagus nerve described above can introduce fun into your journey while also helping to restore joy to your life. Whatever you choose, always remember that your journey is unique to you, and that it can't be compared to anybody else's. Everyone is on their own timeline and everybody is wonderfully unique, so we all have different ways of healing and feeling.

Toning your vagus nerve can be done in many ways, and regardless of whether you want to spend three minutes or thirty minutes a day practicing these different techniques, I don't doubt for a second it'll be worth it.

If you found this book helpful, please leave a review to let us know what you think!

References

Ackerman, C. E. (2019, June 21). *What is self-regulation? (+95 skills and strategies).* PositivePsychology.com. https://positivepsychology.com/self-regulation/

Alcohol Health and Research World. (1997). The principles of nerve cell communication. *Alcohol Health and Research World,* *21*(2), 107–108. https://www.ncbi.nlm.nih.gov/pmc/articles/PMC6826 821/

Alvares, G. A., Quintana, D. S., Hickie, I. B., & Guastella, A. J. (2016). Autonomic nervous system dysfunction in psychiatric disorders and the impact of psychotropic medications: a systematic review and meta-analysis. *Journal of Psychiatry & Neuroscience,* *41*(2), 89–104. https://doi.org/10.1503/jpn.140217

American Headache Society. (2022, June 26). *Vagus nerve stimulation for migraine and cluster headache.* American Headache Society. https://americanheadachesociety.org/news/vagus-nerve-stimulation-for-migraine-and-cluster-headache/

American Psychological Association. (2020, October). *Stress in America 2020: A national mental health crisis.* American Psychological Association; American Psychological Association. https://www.apa.org/news/press/releases/stress/2020/report-october

Anxiety Recovery Centre Victoria. (n.d.). *Vagus nerve exercises.* Anxiety Recovery Centre Victoria. Retrieved September 21, 2022, from https://www.arcvic.org.au/34-resources/402-vagus-nerve-exercises

Apollo. (2022, June 6). Surprising fact! Frequent yawning be a symptom to a health problem. *Apollo 247.* https://www.apollo247.com/blog/article/is-frequent-yawning-a-health-problem

Atlantomed. (2022, March 11). *Vagus nerve disorders.* Atlantomed. https://atlantomed.eu/en/disorders/vagus-nerve-disorders

Banks, D. (2016, April 4). What is brain plasticity and why is it so important? *The Conversation.* https://theconversation.com/what-is-brain-plasticity-and-why-is-it-so-important-55967

Batista, B. (2021, September 14). *The healing benefits of QiGong.* Bodhi Medical QiGong. https://bodhimedicalqigong.com/healing-benefits-of-qigong/

Baxter, S. (n.d.). Somatic meditation to release trauma stored in the body [YouTube Video]. In *YouTube*. Retrieved September 20, 2022, from https://www.youtube.com/watch?v=yCMCKEeG29w

Baxter, S. (2020a). Polyvagal theory explained simply [YouTube Video]. In *YouTube*. https://www.youtube.com/watch?v=OeokFxnhGQo&t=773s

Baxter, S. (2020b). Vagus nerve reset to release trauma stored in the body (Polyvagal exercise) [YouTube Video]. In *YouTube*. https://www.youtube.com/watch?v=eFV0FfMc_uo

Baxter, S. (2020c). Vagus nerve exercises to rewire your brain from anxiety [YouTube Video]. In *YouTube*. https://www.youtube.com/watch?v=L1HCG3BGK8I

Bhattacharya, C. (2018, January 13). *Seven common types of headaches and how to fight them.* Dignity Health. https://www.dignityhealth.org/articles/7-common-types-of-headaches-and-how-to-fight-them

Bolen, B. (2020, January 21). *What triggers the vagal response.* Verywell Health. https://www.verywellhealth.com/vasovagal-reflex-1945072

Borst, S. E., Goswami, S., Lowenthal, D. T., & Newell, D. (2007). Autonomic nervous system. *Encyclopedia of Gerontology*, 129–135. https://doi.org/10.1016/b0-12-370870-2/00019-6

Brain Harmony. (2020, September 20). *How vagal regulation impacts chronic fatigue syndrome.* Brain Harmony. https://www.brainharmony.com/blog/2020/9/20/how-vagal-regulation-impacts-chronic-fatigue-

syndrome#:~:text=A%20growing%20amount%20of%
20research

Breit, S., Kupferberg, A., Rogler, G., & Hasler, G. (2018).
Vagus nerve as modulator of the brain-gut axis in
psychiatric and inflammatory disorders. *Frontiers in
Psychiatry*, *9*(44).
https://doi.org/10.3389/fpsyt.2018.00044

Caffrey, J. (2019, November 18). How to access the vagus
nerve with cold water. *Justin Caffrey*.
https://www.justincaffrey.com/my-
blog/2019/3/6/cold-water-and-the-vagus-nerve

Caffrey, J. (2021). Game changing vagus nerve exercise
(parasympathetic shift) [YouTube Video]. In *YouTube*.
https://www.youtube.com/clip/UgkxVfOkwwOdX1e
GP8PPEJfPaULzwt30LfYK

Campos, M. (2021, December 1). Heart rate variability: A new
way to track well-being. *Harvard Health*.
https://www.health.harvard.edu/blog/heart-rate-
variability-new-way-track-well-2017112212789

Capozzi, B. (2020, December 18). *Exploring the "Vagus" Strip:
Why the Vagus Nerve is Key to Mental Health*. Step up for
Mental Health.
https://www.stepupformentalhealth.org/exploring-the-
vagus-strip-why-the-vagus-nerve-is-key-to-mental-
health/

Case-Lo, C. (2019, March 8). *Autonomic dysfunction*. Healthline.
https://www.healthline.com/health/autonomic-
dysfunction

Centeno, C. (2020, January 13). The vagus nerve, neck pain,
anxiety, headaches, and depression. *Regenexx*.

https://regenexx.com/blog/vagus-nerve-and-neck-pain/

Centers for Disease Control and Prevention. (2020, May 19). *High blood pressure: About high blood pressure.* Centers for Disease Control and Prevention. https://www.cdc.gov/bloodpressure/about.htm#:~:te xt=High%20blood%20pressure%20can%20damage%2 0your%20arteries%20by%20making%20them

Chapleau, M. W., & Sabharwal, R. (2011). Methods of assessing vagus nerve activity and reflexes. *Heart Failure Reviews, 16*(2), 109–127. https://doi.org/10.1007/s10741-010-9174-6

Cherry, K. (2022, September 22). *What is mindfulness meditation?* Verywellmind; Verywellmind. https://www.verywellmind.com/mindfulness-meditation-88369

Clarke, J. (2019). *Polyvagal theory and how it relates to social cues.* Verywell Mind. https://www.verywellmind.com/polyvagal-theory-4588049

Cleveland Clinic. (n.d.-a). *Diaphragm.* Cleveland Clinic. Retrieved September 22, 2022, from https://my.clevelandclinic.org/health/body/21578-diaphragm#:~:text=The%20diaphragm%20is%20a%20 muscle%20that%20helps%20you%20inhale%20and

Cleveland Clinic. (n.d.-b). *Fatigue.* Cleveland Clinic. Retrieved September 22, 2022, from https://my.clevelandclinic.org/health/symptoms/2120 6-fatigue#:~:text=Fatigue%20is%20feeling%20severely% 20overtired

Cleveland Clinic. (n.d.-c). *Uvula.* Cleveland Clinic. Retrieved September 27, 2022, from https://my.clevelandclinic.org/health/body/22674-uvula

Cleveland Clinic. (2020a, May 29). *Cryotherapy.* Cleveland Clinic. https://my.clevelandclinic.org/health/treatments/21099-cryotherapy

Cleveland Clinic. (2020b, September 24). *Irritable bowel syndrome (IBS).* Cleveland Clinic. https://my.clevelandclinic.org/health/diseases/4342-irritable-bowel-syndrome-ibs

Cleveland Clinic. (2020c, December 5). *Nervous system.* Cleveland Clinic. https://my.clevelandclinic.org/health/articles/21202-nervous-system#:~:text=Your%20nervous%20system%20is%20your

Cleveland Clinic. (2021a, July 28). *Inflammation.* Cleveland Clinic. https://my.clevelandclinic.org/health/symptoms/21660-inflammation

Cleveland Clinic. (2021b, October 8). *Oculomotor nerve.* Cleveland Clinic. https://my.clevelandclinic.org/health/body/21708-oculomotor-nerve#:~:text=like%20your%20eyes.-

Cleveland Clinic. (2021c, December 29). *Facial nerve.* Cleveland Clinic. https://my.clevelandclinic.org/health/body/22218-facial-nerve#:~:text=What%20is%20the%20facial%20nerve

Cleveland Clinic. (2022a, January 11). *Glossopharyngeal nerve.* Cleveland Clinic. https://my.clevelandclinic.org/health/body/22269-glossopharyngeal-nerve#:~:text=Part%20of%20the%20tongue%3A%20The

Cleveland Clinic. (2022b, January 11). *Vagus nerve.* Cleveland Clinic. https://my.clevelandclinic.org/health/body/22279-vagus-nerve#:~:text=What%20is%20the%20Vagus%20Nerve

Cleveland Clinic. (2022c, March 10). *Five ways to stimulate your vagus nerve: The longest cranial nerve in your body plays a role in your health.* Cleveland Clinic. https://health.clevelandclinic.org/vagus-nerve-stimulation/

Cleveland Clinic. (2022d, March 22). *Nerves.* Cleveland Clinic. https://my.clevelandclinic.org/health/body/22584-nerves

Cooper, M. (2021, April 21). We tried it: Wim Hof's 20-day cold shower challenge. *Artful Living.* https://artfulliving.com/we-tried-it-wim-hof-cold-water-challenge-review/

Costa, M., Brookes, S. J. H., & Hennig, G. W. (2000). Anatomy and physiology of the enteric nervous system. *Gut, 47*(90004), 15iv19. https://doi.org/10.1136/gut.47.suppl_4.iv15

Course Hero, Inc. (2022). *The nervous system.* CliffsNotes; Course Hero, Inc. https://www.cliffsnotes.com/study-guides/anatomy-and-physiology/the-nervous-system/nervous-system-terminology

Crist, C. (2022, February 15). *Long COVID symptoms linked to effects on vagus nerve.* WebMD. https://www.webmd.com/lung/news/20220215/covid-symptoms-linked-to-vagus-nerve

Cronkleton, E. (2021, February 11). *Face yoga for inner and outer radiance?* Healthline. https://www.healthline.com/health/fitness-exercise/face-yoga#takeaway

Cuevas, J. (2015). The somatic nervous system. *XPharm: The Comprehensive Pharmacology Reference*, 1–13. https://doi.org/10.1016/b978-0-12-801238-3.05364-2

Cuncic, A. (2022, January 27). *How to develop and practice self-regulation.* Verywell Mind. https://www.verywellmind.com/how-you-can-practice-self-regulation-4163536#:~:text=Self%2Dregulation%20is%20the%20ability

Daily Calm. (2016). 10 minute mindfulness meditation: Be present [YouTube Video]. In *YouTube.* https://www.youtube.com/watch?v=ZToicYcHIOU

David Zelman. (2020). *What Is inflammation?* WebMD; WebMD. https://www.webmd.com/arthritis/about-inflammation

Davidson, K. (2021, February 11). *QiGong meditation techniques: Benefits and how to do it.* Healthline. https://www.healthline.com/nutrition/qigong-meditation#types

De Ridder, D., Langguth, B., & Vanneste, S. (2021). Vagus nerve stimulation for tinnitus: A review and perspective. *Progress in Brain Research, 262,* 451–467. https://doi.org/10.1016/bs.pbr.2020.08.011

Elgot, J. (2015, July 13). Gwyneth Paltrow's guide to yawning. *The Guardian.* https://www.theguardian.com/science/2015/jul/13/g wyneth-paltrows-guide-to-yawning

Epstein, O. (2021, July 15). *Vagus nerve dysfunction: what it is and what are the main symptoms?* Top Doctors. https://www.topdoctors.co.uk/medical-articles/vagus-nerve-dysfunction-what-is-it-and-what-are-the-main-symptoms#

Erman, A., Kejner, A., Hogikyan, N., & Feldman, E. (2009). Disorders of cranial nerves IX and X. *Seminars in Neurology, 29*(01), 085–092. https://doi.org/10.1055/s-0028-1124027

Eunice Kennedy Shriver National Institute of Child Health and Human Development. (n.d.). *What are the parts of the nervous system?* National Institute of Child Health and Human Development. Retrieved September 12, 2022, from https://www.nichd.nih.gov/health/topics/neuro/cond itioninfo/parts#

Fallis, J. (2017). *How to stimulate your vagus nerve for better mental health.* https://sass.uottawa.ca/sites/sass.uottawa.ca/files/how _to_stimulate_your_vagus_nerve_for_better_mental_h ealth_1.pdf

Fisher, S. (2019, November 27). Work life balance: What does it mean and why does it matter? *Qualtrics XM.* https://www.qualtrics.com/blog/work-life-balance/

Fitzgerald, J. (2019, January 22). *The difference between depression and sadness.* Medical News Today. https://www.medicalnewstoday.com/articles/314418# knowing-the-difference

Flatirons Integrative Health & Nutrition. (n.d.). *Vagus nerve dysfunction*. Flatirons Integrative Health & Nutrition; Squarespace. Retrieved September 15, 2022, from https://www.flatironsintegrative.com/vagusnerve

Frank, M. (2022, August 12). *Can't get anything done? Why ADHD brains become paralyzed in quarantine*. ADDitude. https://www.additudemag.com/polyvagal-theory-adhd-brain-cant-get-anything-done/

Frothingham, S. (2019, December 18). *Benefits of ujjayi breathing and how to do it*. Healthline. https://www.healthline.com/health/fitness-exercise/ujjayi-breathing

Geddes, L. (2013, August 14). *Head hurts? Zap the wonder nerve in your neck*. New Scientist. https://www.newscientist.com/article/mg21929303-200-head-hurts-zap-the-wonder-nerve-in-your-neck/

Gelles, D. (n.d.). *How to meditate*. The New York Times. Retrieved September 29, 2022, from https://www.nytimes.com/guides/well/how-to-meditate#:~:text=Mindfulness%20meditation%20is%20the%20practice%20of%20actually%20being%20present%20in

Gernon, D. (2019, May 28). *On knowing the difference between sadness and depression*. A Lust for Life. https://www.alustforlife.com/tools/mental-health/on-knowing-the-difference-between-sadness-and-depression?gclid=Cj0KCQjwj7CZBhDHARIsAPPWv3e9T69lCylDivF1aO2KYtS3ePCUfTDb29gPj0q6qIjXlcAaMrlmSAYaAo9DEALw_wcB

Gotter, A. (2020, March 2). *Benefits of cryotherapy*. Healthline. https://www.healthline.com/health/cryotherapy-benefits#risks-and-side-effects

Gould, K. (2019, November 12). *The vagus nerve: Your body's communication superhighway.* Live Science; Live Science. https://www.livescience.com/vagus-nerve.html

Greenawald, E. (2021, September 21). *Ten types of journaling for peace of mind.* Skillshare Blog. https://www.skillshare.com/blog/10-types-of-journaling-for-peace-of-mind/

Greene, C. (n.d.). How to laugh more alone [YouTube Video]. In *YouTube.* Retrieved September 27, 2022, from https://www.youtube.com/watch?v=TGVcxENdAeo

Harvard Health. (2022, May 24). *The health benefits of tai chi.* Harvard Health; Harvard Health Publishing. https://www.health.harvard.edu/staying-healthy/the-health-benefits-of-tai-chi

Hauser, R. (2022). *Vagus nerve compression in the neck: Symptoms and treatments – Caring Medical Florida.* Caring Medical. https://www.caringmedical.com/prolotherapy-news/vagus-nerve-compression-cervical-spine/

healthessentials. (2021, June 14). *Why Gua Sha might be good for you: Find out what it is and how it can help the body heal.* Cleveland Clinic. https://health.clevelandclinic.org/why-gua-sha-might-be-good-for-you/

Henssen, D. J. H. A., Derks, B., Van Doorn, M., Verhoogt, N., Van Cappellen van Walsum, A.-M., Staats, P., & Vissers, K. (2019). Vagus nerve stimulation for primary headache disorders: An anatomical review to explain a clinical phenomenon. *Cephalalgia, 39*(9), 1180–1194. https://doi.org/10.1177/0333102419833076

Higuera, V. (2017, June 14). *Six possible causes of brain fog.* Healthline; Healthline Media. https://www.healthline.com/health/brain-fog

Ho, T. C., & King, L. S. (2021). Mechanisms of neuroplasticity linking early adversity to depression: developmental considerations. *Translational Psychiatry, 11*(1), 1–13. https://doi.org/10.1038/s41398-021-01639-6

Horeis, M. (2020, June 23). *The vagus nerve: Your secret weapon in fighting stress.* Allied Services Integrated Health System. https://www.allied-services.org/news/2020/june/the-vagus-nerve-your-secret-weapon-in-fighting-s/

Huzar, T. (2021, July 7). *What is the difference between IBS and IBD?* Medical News Today. https://www.medicalnewstoday.com/articles/323778#takeaway

Indwell Counseling. (2019, June 11). *The vagus nerve: Becoming unfrozen.* Indwell Counseling. https://www.indwellcounseling.com/blog/blog-5

Integrative Bodywork. (2018, July 7). *Five minutes to freeing up vagus nerve.* Integrative Bodywork. https://integrativebodyworkclaremont.com/blogposts/five-minutes-to-freeing-up-vagus-nerve

Iron Neck. (2021, October 4). *Vagus nerve and pain in the neck: Diagnosis and treatment.* Iron Neck. https://www.iron-neck.com/blogs/news/vagus-nerve-pain

Ishler, J. (2021, September 16). *How to release "emotional baggage" and the tension that goes with it.* Healthline. https://www.healthline.com/health/mind-body/how-to-release-emotional-baggage-and-the-tension-that-goes-with-it

Jacob, D. (2020, October 15). *Can the vagus nerve cause seizures?* MedicineNet. https://www.medicinenet.com/can_the_vagus_nerve_cause_seizures/article.htm

Jefferson, B. (2021, December 7). *How do others help us regulate emotions?* Neuroscience News.com. https://neurosciencenews.com/supportive-emotional-regulation-19764/

Joyce, C., Le, P. H., & Peterson, D. C. (2019, August 14). *Neuroanatomy, cranial nerve 3 (Oculomotor).* National Library of Medicine; StatPearls Publishing. https://www.ncbi.nlm.nih.gov/books/NBK537126/

Kent, X. (2017, March 7). *Ten vagus nerve symptoms and how to treat them.* GetZoneDup. http://getzonedup.com/vagus-nerve-symptoms/

Khalsa, P. (n.d.). *About yogi Bhajan and kundalini yoga.* Kundalini Yoga; 3HO Foundation. Retrieved September 29, 2022, from http://www.kundaliniyoga.co.za/kundalini-yoga/about-yogi-bhajan/

Killeen, J. (2020, June 17). *Learn about the health impacts of orgasms!* Avant Gynecology. https://www.avantgynecology.com/2020/06/17/learn-about-the-health-impacts-of-orgasms/

Knight, E. L., Giuliano, R. J., Shank, S. W., Clarke, M. M., & Almeida, D. M. (2020). Parasympathetic and sympathetic nervous systems interactively predict change in cognitive functioning in midlife adults. *Psychophysiology, 57*(10). https://doi.org/10.1111/psyp.13622

Kurosu, C., & Kuhn, A. (2019, February 15). *Qigong and Tai Chi benefits.* YMAA.

https://ymaa.com/articles/2018/11/qigong-and-tai-chi-benefits

Lakna. (2017, August 1). *Difference between cranial and spinal nerves.* PEDIAA. https://pediaa.com/difference-between-cranial-and-spinal-nerves/

Lam, P. (2018). *What is Tai chi and what are the health benefits?* Tai Chi for Health Institute. https://taichiforhealthinstitute.org/what-is-tai-chi/

Lanese, N., & Dutfield, S. (2022, February 9). *Fight or flight: The sympathetic nervous system.* Live Science; Live Science. https://www.livescience.com/65446-sympathetic-nervous-system.html

Larkin, B. (n.d.). Kundalini yoga for beginners: How to do breath of fire tutorial [YouTube Video]. In *YouTube.* Retrieved September 20, 2022, from https://www.youtube.com/watch?v=SQS4Ad-16vE

LaughActive. (n.d.). How to laugh more alone [YouTube Video]. In *YouTube.* Retrieved September 26, 2022, from https://www.youtube.com/watch?v=TGVcxENdAeo

lcviweb. (2020, March 12). *Laughter yoga alone for you.* Laughter Clubs Victo. https://www.laughterclubsvic.org.au/post/laughter-yoga-alone-for-you

Leber, J. (2014, January 6). *An atlas of the human body that maps where we feel emotions.* Fast Company. https://www.fastcompany.com/3024327/an-atlas-of-the-human-body-that-maps-where-we-feel-emotions#:~:text=Happiness%20uses%20your%20whole%20body

Lee, L. (2022, August 19). *How to diagnose vagus nerve damage: A complete guide to the symptoms of gastroparesis and getting diagnosed.* WikiHow. https://www.wikihow.com/Diagnose-Vagus-Nerve-Damage

Low, P. (2019). *Overview of the autonomic nervous system.* Merck Manuals Consumer Version. https://www.merckmanuals.com/home/brain

Low, P. (2020, April). *Overview of the autonomic nervous system.* MSD Manual Consumer Version. https://www.msdmanuals.com/home/brain

Low, P. (2021, September). *Autonomic neuropathies.* Merck Manuals Consumer Version. https://www.merckmanuals.com/home/brain

Lyon, B. (2016, January 12). *Anatomy of a freeze - or dorsal vagal shutdown.* Center for Healing Shame. https://healingshame.com/articles/anatomy-of-a-freeze-or-dorsal-vagal-shutdown-bret-lyon-phd

Maguire, J. (2021, October 14). *You can't out-think your feelings when you're triggered.* Jessica Maguire. https://www.jessicamaguire.com/resources/2021/10/14/why-the-vagus-nerve-reduces-anxiety

Mallenbaum, C., Rivas, A., & Goldberg, E. (2022, March 3). *Does vagus nerve icing really help with anxiety? We asked an expert.* The Skimm'. https://www.theskimm.com/wellness/vagus-nerve-stimulation-anxiety

Mark. (2021, July 10). *The five best sternocleidomastoid stretches.* Posture Direct. https://www.posturedirect.com/sternocleidomastoid-stretches/

Mateos-Aparicio, P., & Rodríguez-Moreno, A. (2019). The impact of studying brain plasticity. *Frontiers in Cellular Neuroscience, 13*(66). https://doi.org/10.3389/fncel.2019.00066

May, L. (2020, May 6). *Somatic mindfulness exercises and treatment from anywhere.* Trauma and beyond Psychological Center. https://www.traumaandbeyondcenter.com/blog/somat ic-mindfulness-exercises-and-treatment-from-anywhere/

Mayo Clinic. (n.d.-a). *Anxiety disorders.* Mayo Clinic. Retrieved September 23, 2022, from https://www.mayoclinic.org/diseases-conditions/anxiety/symptoms-causes/syc-20350961#:~:text=Panic%20disorder%20involves%20 repeated%20episodes

Mayo Clinic. (n.d.-b). *Hyperthyroidism (overactive thyroid).* Mayo Clinic. Retrieved September 19, 2022, from https://www.mayoclinic.org/diseases-conditions/hyperthyroidism/symptoms-causes/syc-20373659#:~:text=Overview

Mayo Clinic. (n.d.-c). *Thyroid cancer.* Mayo Clinic. Retrieved September 19, 2022, from https://www.mayoclinic.org/diseases-conditions/thyroid-cancer/symptoms-causes/syc-20354161#:~:text=The%20thyroid%20is%20a%20butt erfly

Mayo Clinic. (2016, October 15). *Insomnia.* Mayo Clinic. https://www.mayoclinic.org/diseases-conditions/insomnia/symptoms-causes/syc-20355167

Mayo Clinic. (2017). *Bruxism (teeth grinding).* Mayo Clinic. https://www.mayoclinic.org/diseases-conditions/bruxism/symptoms-causes/syc-20356095

Mayo Clinic. (2018a). *Autonomic neuropathy: Symptoms and causes.* Mayo Clinic. https://www.mayoclinic.org/diseases-conditions/autonomic-neuropathy/symptoms-causes/syc-20369829

Mayo Clinic. (2018b). *Tinnitus.* Mayo Clinic. https://www.mayoclinic.org/diseases-conditions/tinnitus/symptoms-causes/syc-20350156

Mayo Clinic. (2018c). *TMJ disorders.* Mayo Clinic. https://www.mayoclinic.org/diseases-conditions/tmj/symptoms-causes/syc-20350941

Mayo Clinic. (2018d). *Vasovagal syncope.* Mayo Clinic. https://www.mayoclinic.org/diseases-conditions/vasovagal-syncope/symptoms-causes/syc-20350527

Mayo Clinic. (2020a). *Hypothyroidism (underactive thyroid).* Mayo Clinic. https://www.mayoclinic.org/diseases-conditions/hypothyroidism/symptoms-causes/syc-20350284

Mayo Clinic. (2020b). *Peptic ulcer.* Mayo Clinic. https://www.mayoclinic.org/diseases-conditions/peptic-ulcer/symptoms-causes/syc-20354223

Mayo Foundation for Medical Education and Research. (2022). *Low blood pressure (hypotension).* Mayo Clinic. https://www.mayoclinic.org/diseases-conditions/low-blood-pressure/symptoms-causes/syc-20355465

McLaughlin, K. A., Rith-Najarian, L., Dirks, M. A., & Sheridan, M. A. (2013). Low vagal tone magnifies the association between psychosocial stress exposure and internalizing psychopathology in adolescents. *Journal of Clinical Child*

      *   Adolescent   Psychology*,   *44*(2),   314–328. https://doi.org/10.1080/15374416.2013.843464

Mehmed, S. E. (2015). Effect of vagal stimulation in acute asthma. *Clinical and Translational Allergy*, *5*(S2). https://doi.org/10.1186/2045-7022-5-s2-p13

Meridian Senior Living. (2021, September 8). Five benefits of social engagement for seniors. *Meridian Senior Living.* https://www.meridiansenior.com/blog/five-benefits-of-social-engagement-for-seniors#:~:text=Being%20socially%20active%20can%20have

Messina, I., Calvo, V., Masaro, C., Ghedin, S., & Marogna, C. (2021). Interpersonal emotion: From R=research to group therapy. *Frontiers in Psychology*, *12.* https://doi.org/10.3389/fpsyg.2021.636919

Metabolic Meals. (2021, June 20). A beginner's guide to heart rate variability (HRV). *Metabolic Meals.* https://blog.mymetabolicmeals.com/hrv-guide/

Migala, J. (2021a, June 23). How to stimulate the vagus nerve: 8 exercises to try for calm. *Parsley Health.* https://www.parsleyhealth.com/blog/how-to-stimulate-vagus-nerve-exercises/

Migala, J. (2021b, June 23). *Vagus nerve stimulation: Eight exercises to try for calm.* Parsley Health. https://www.parsleyhealth.com/blog/how-to-stimulate-vagus-nerve-exercises/#:~:text=Deep%20breathing%3A%20The%20Box%20Breath

Miller, J. (n.d.). Hum to activate the vagus nerve [YouTube Video]. In *YouTube.* Retrieved September 21, 2022,

from
https://www.youtube.com/watch?v=QSAvPgqQ2L0

Miller, J. (2022). A vagus nerve myofascial self-massage for downregulation [YouTube Video]. In *YouTube*. https://www.youtube.com/watch?v=ag3SQBFHKes

Mind. (2018, July). *Why do I get angry?* Mind. https://www.mind.org.uk/information-support/types-of-mental-health-problems/anger/causes-of-anger/#:~:text=Everyone%20has%20their%20own%20Otriggers

Mindmadeeasy. (n.d.). What is the polyvagal theory? [YouTube Video]. In *YouTube*. Retrieved May 30, 2022, from https://www.youtube.com/watch?v=zYvZUorQbrg

Missimer, A. (2021a, January 25). *How to test your vagus nerve: Polyvagal theory.* The Movement Paradigm. https://themovementparadigm.com/how-to-test-your-vagus-nerve/

Missimer, A. (2021b, February 13). *How to map your nervous system: The polyvagal theory.* The Movement Paradigm. https://themovementparadigm.com/category/blog/physical-therapy/

Missimer, A. (2021c). The trap squeeze test (by Stanley Rosenberg) [Facebook Video]. In *Crazy Ebook*. https://m.facebook.com/themovementparadigm/videos/the-trap-squeeze-test-by-stanley-rosenberg-is-a-great-and-simple-way-to-test-the/937446390374907/?_rdr

Missimer, A. (2021d, December 16). *Vagus nerve hack: Trapezius twist.* The Movement Paradigm. https://themovementparadigm.com/trapezius-twist/

Missimer, A. (2022, January 27). *Jaw-Emotion Link*. The Movement Paradigm. https://themovementparadigm.com/jaw-emotion-link/

Murray, N. (2017, May 9). *The healing capacity of the vagus nerve*. Botanica Health. https://www.botanicahealth.co.uk/the-healing-capacity-of-the-vagus-nerve/

MyHealthFinder. (2022, July 20). *Health conditions: Manage stress*. MyHealthFinder; Office of Disease Prevention and Health Promotion. https://health.gov/myhealthfinder/health-conditions/heart-health/manage-stress

N. (2018, September 9). *Vagus nerve: A path to healing*. The Holistic Psychologist. https://theholisticpsychologist.com/vagus_nerve_a_path-to-healing/

National Alliance On Mental Illness. (2020). *Depression*. National Alliance on Mental Illness. https://www.nami.org/About-Mental-Illness/Mental-Health-Conditions/Depression

National Alliance on Mental Illness. (2017). *Anxiety disorders*. National Alliance on Mental Illness. https://www.nami.org/About-Mental-Illness/Mental-Health-Conditions/Anxiety-Disorders

National Cancer Institute. (2011, February 2). *Spinal cord*. NCI's Dictionary of Cancer Terms. https://www.cancer.gov/publications/dictionaries/cancer-terms/def/spinal-cord

National Cancer Institute. (2019). Review: Introduction to the nervous system. In *SEER Training Modules*. Surveillance, Epidemiology and End Results Program.

https://training.seer.cancer.gov/anatomy/nervous/revi
ew.html

National Center for Biotechnology Information. (2020, April
23). *How does the immune system work?* National Library of
Medicine; Institute for Quality and Efficiency in Health
Care   (IQWiG).
https://www.ncbi.nlm.nih.gov/books/NBK279364/

National Institute on Alcohol Abuse and Alcoholism. (1997).
The principles of nerve cell communication. *Alcohol
Health and Research World, 21*(2), 107–108.
https://www.ncbi.nlm.nih.gov/pmc/articles/PMC6826
821/

Nemechek, P. (2016, November 6). *Brain fog.* Nemechek
Autonomic   Medicine.
https://www.nemechekconsultativemedicine.com/blog
/brain-fog/

NeuroLife. (2022). *Acute and structural pain/conditions.* NeuroLife
Chiropractic and Functional Medicine Center.
https://www.neurolifecenter.com/specialities/acute-
and-structural-pain-conditions/

Neuvana. (2020, April 13). *Vagus nerve science for a better night's
sleep.*   Neuvana.
https://neuvanalife.com/blogs/blog/vagus-nerve-
science-for-a-better-nights-sleep

Noble, L. J., Souza, R. R., & McIntyre, C. K. (2018). Vagus
nerve stimulation as a tool for enhancing extinction in
exposure-based therapies. *Psychopharmacology, 236*(1).
https://doi.org/10.1007/s00213-018-4994-5

Nunez, K. (2020a, February 21). *Fight, fight, freeze: What this
response means.* Healthline.

https://www.healthline.com/health/mental-health/fight-flight-freeze#:~:text=It

Nunez, K. (2020b, July 16). *What is kundalini yoga and what are the benefits?* Healthline. https://www.healthline.com/health/kundalini-yoga

Nurse Linda. (2022, February 16). *The vagus nerve.* Christopher & Dana Reeve Foundation; Life After Paralysis. https://www.christopherreeve.org/blog/life-after-paralysis/the-vagus-nerve

Ogle, K. T. (2012). Is your patient having a vasovagal reaction? *Nursing Made Incredibly Easy!, 10*(3), 56. https://doi.org/10.1097/01.nme.0000413348.75316.a0

Paltrow, G. (n.d.). *Why yawning is important - and how to optimize the reflex.* Goop. Retrieved September 26, 2022, from https://goop.com/wellness/health/why-yawning-is-important-and-how-to-optimize-the-reflex/

Patterson, E. (2022, September 5). *Stress facts and statistics.* The Recovery Village. https://www.therecoveryvillage.com/mental-health/stress/stress-statistics/#:~:text=Statistics%20demonstrate%20the%20widespread%20prevalence

People's Center. (2021, May 11). *Stressed? You should learn more about this chemical.* People's Center Clinics & Services. https://www.peoples-center.org/blog/stress#:~:text=The%20two%20chemicals%20released%20by

Perros, P., Hunter, J., & Strachan, M. (n.d.). *Hair loss and thyroid disorders.* British Thyroid Foundation. Retrieved September 19, 2022, from https://www.btf-thyroid.org/hair-loss-and-thyroid-

disorders#:~:text=Severe%20and%20prolonged%20hy
pothyroidism%20and

Peter, S., & Burcham, C. (2022, August 26). *This is exactly how to use your Gua Sha face tool.* Byrdie. https://www.byrdie.com/gua-sha

Physiopedia. (2022a). *Parasympathetic system.* Physiopedia. https://www.physio-pedia.com/Parasympathetic_System

Physiopedia. (2022b). *Vagus nerve.* Physiopedia. https://www.physio-pedia.com/Vagus_Nerve#:~:text=The%20vagus%20nerve%20runs%20from

Piedmont. (2022). *The difference between tai chi and qi gong.* Piedmont. https://www.piedmont.org/living-better/the-difference-between-tai-chi-and-qi-gong

Porges, S. W. (2022). *Home of Dr. Stephen Porges.* Stephen W. Porges, PhD. https://www.stephenporges.com/

PsychAlive. (2018). Dr. Stephen Porges: What is the polyvagal theory [YouTube Video]. In *YouTube.* https://www.youtube.com/watch?v=ec3AUMDjtKQ&t=2s

Psychology Today. (n.d.). *Vagus nerve.* Psychology Today. Retrieved September 13, 2022, from https://www.psychologytoday.com/us/basics/vagus-nerve

Raypole, C. (2020, August 18). *Have trouble meditating? Try mantra meditation.* Healthline. https://www.healthline.com/health/mantra-meditation#how-to

Rea, P. (2014). Introduction to the nervous system. *Clinical Anatomy of the Cranial Nerves*, xv–xxix. https://doi.org/10.1016/b978-0-12-800898-0.00019-1

Regional Neurological Associates. (2020, August 17). *What do the different parts of the nervous system do?* Regional Neurological Associates. https://www.regionalneurological.com/parts-of-the-nervous-system/

Reid, M. (2018, July 10). *Can tinnitus be cured? Here's what the latest research says.* Everyday Health. https://www.everydayhealth.com/tinnitus/can-tinnitus-cured-heres-what-latest-research-says/

Robertson, R. (2020, August 20). *The gut-brain connection: How it works and the role of nutrition.* Healthline. https://www.healthline.com/nutrition/gut-brain-connection#TOC_TITLE_HDR_2

Rosenberg, S. (2019). *Accessing the healing power of the vagus nerve: Self-help exercises for anxiety, depression, trauma, and autism.* Readhowyouwant Com Ltd.

Rubin, M. (2020, April). *Overview of the peripheral nervous system.* MSD Manual Consumer Version. https://www.msdmanuals.com/home/brain

Rukmani, M. R., Seshadri, S. P., Thennarasu, K., Raju, T. R., & Sathyaprabha, T. N. (2016). Heart rate variability in children with Attention-Deficit/Hyperactivity Disorder: A pilot study. *Annals of Neurosciences, 23*(2), 81–88. https://doi.org/10.1159/000443574

Ruscio, M. (2022, January 10). What Is Vagal Tone and How to Improve Yours. *Dr. Ruscio.* https://drruscio.com/vagal-tone/

Sarmadi, R. (2019, June 18). *Does cryotherapy activate the vagus nerve?* Cryo Innovations. https://www.cryoinnovations.com/blog/2019/6/18/vagnus-nerve-activation-through-cryotherapy#.YzFq6HZBy3A

Schick, H. (2018, May 2). Thyroid Disorders [Interview]. In *HighPoint Health Center.* https://www.highpointhealth.com/thyroid-disorders-podcast/

Schwartz, A. (n.d.-a). Mini yoga flow: Engaging the vagus nerve [YouTube Video]. In *YouTube.* Retrieved September 21, 2022, from https://www.youtube.com/watch?v=WkjAbgEw_F8

Schwartz, A. (n.d.-b). Nervous system support: Eye movement, courage, and your vagus nerve [YouTube Video]. In *YouTube.* Retrieved September 21, 2022, from https://www.youtube.com/watch?v=cxFvnsqxb70

Schwartz, A. (n.d.-c). Vagus nerve and fascia release for the diaphragm: Balls, straps, and rollers [YouTube Video]. In *YouTube.* Retrieved September 21, 2022, from https://www.youtube.com/watch?v=SMrM0jrYjUU

Schwartz, A. (2020, July 1). The vagus nerve and your health. *Dr Arielle Schwartz.* https://drarielleschwartz.com/the-vagus-nerve-and-your-health-dr-arielle-schwartz/#.YysCzHZBy3B

Schwartz, A. (2021, September 16). *The vagus nerve and eye movements: Tools for trauma recovery.* Dr Arielle Schwartz. https://drarielleschwartz.com/the-vagus-nerve-and-eye-movements-tools-for-trauma-recovery-dr-arielle-schwartz/#.YysEU3ZBy3B

Schwartz, A. (2022, May 2). *Fascia and the vagus nerve: Heling from the inside out.* YogaUOnline.com. https://yogauonline.com/yoga-for-stress-relief/fascia-and-vagus-nerve-healing-inside-out

Seladi-Schulman, J. (2022, July 22). *What is the vagus nerve?* Healthline. https://www.healthline.com/human-body-maps/vagus-nerve#other-considerations

Shah, A. (2021, January). *Is my anxiety, stress and tiredness linked with my TMJ disorder?* TMJ, Tongue Tie & Sleep Institute; Tongue Tie India. https://www.tonguetieindia.com/is-my-anxiety-stress-and-tiredness-linked-with-my-tmj-disorder.html

Shah, S. (2021, March 29). *Seven common ways of vagus nerve stimulation to nourish your body and mind.* The Art of Living. https://www.artofliving.org/us-en/7-natural-ways-to-strengthen-and-stimulate-your-vagus-nerve-today

Silverstein, E. (2017, January 13). *Vagus nerve and tears.* On Sticky Topics. https://onstickytopics.com/2017/01/vagus-nerve-tears/

Singh Bisht, J. (2011). Very good very good yay! [YouTube Video]. In *YouTube.* https://www.youtube.com/watch?v=Q3hxnXmWot8

Stuart, A. (2021, October 31). *Acupressure points and massage treatment.* WebMD. https://www.webmd.com/balance/guide/acupressure-points-and-massage-treatment

Sunseri, J. (2020, December 22). *Why your vagal brake strength is important.* Justin LMFT. https://www.justinlmft.com/post/why-your-vagal-brake-strength-is-important

Synctuition. (2020, February 27). Healthy body, healthy mind: Six ways to boost your well-being. *Synctuition.* https://synctuition.com/blog/healthy-body-healthy-mind-6-ways-to-boost-your-well-being/#:~:text=As%20the%20adage%20goes%2C%20a

Tarlton, A. (2018, March 16). *What is kundalini yoga? Everything you need to know about this celebrity-favorite practice.* Mindbodygreen. https://www.mindbodygreen.com/articles/kundalini-yoga-101-everything-you-wanted-to-know

The Movement Paradigm. (n.d.-a). How to test your vagus nerve: Polyvagal theory [YouTube Video]. In *YouTube.* Retrieved September 23, 2022, from https://www.youtube.com/watch?v=ukrCgQR5LjY

The Movement Paradigm. (n.d.-b). Vagus Nerve Hack | Cold Water [YouTube Video]. In *YouTube.* Retrieved September 21, 2022, from https://www.youtube.com/watch?v=si1msrS-2oY

Tune Up Fitness. (n.d.). Fascia facial massage for relaxation [YouTube Video]. In *YouTube.* Retrieved September 21, 2022, from https://www.youtube.com/watch?v=wQyX_Dw3lU8

Turner, S. (2021, February 4). *Is the vagus nerve a key to our mental health?* Patient. https://patient.info/news-and-features/is-the-vagus-nerve-really-the-key-to-our-mental-health-and-well-being#:~:text=A%20low%20vagal%20tone%20means

University of Michigan Health. (n.d.). *Diaphragmatic breathing for GI patients.* University of Michigan Health; University of Michigan. Retrieved September 22, 2022, from https://www.uofmhealth.org/conditions-

treatments/digestive-and-liver-health/diaphragmatic-
breathing-gi-patients

University of Rochester Medical Center. (2018). *Neurology at
Highland Hospital: What is a neurologist?* University of
Rochester Medicine.
https://www.urmc.rochester.edu/highland/department
s-centers/neurology/what-is-a-neurologist.aspx

Valenstein, E. S. (2002). The discovery of chemical
neurotransmitters. *Brain and Cognition, 49*(1), 73–95.
https://doi.org/10.1006/brcg.2001.1487

Vann, M. R. (2017, November 6). *Seven healthy reasons you should
have sex - right now!* EverydayHealth.
https://www.everydayhealth.com/sexual-health/seven-
healthy-reasons-to-have-sex-right-now.aspx

Villines, Z. (2020, February 24). *What to know about
sternocleidomastoid pain.* MedicalNewsToday.
https://www.medicalnewstoday.com/articles/sternocle
idomastoid-pain

Wagner, D. (2016, June 27). *Polyvagal theory in practice.*
Counseling Today.
https://ct.counseling.org/2016/06/polyvagal-theory-
practice/

Walinga, J., & Stangor, C. (2014). 4.4 Putting it all together: The
nervous system and the endocrine system. In *Introduction
to psychology: 1st Canadian edition.* Pressbooks.
https://opentextbc.ca/introductiontopsychology/chapt
er/3-4-putting-it-all-together-the-nervous-system-and-
the-endocrine-
system/#:~:text=The%20CNS%20is%20made%20up

Warren, S. (2020, November 16). *How to make meditation part of
your daily life.* Somatic Movement Center.

https://somaticmovementcenter.com/how-to-meditate/#:~:text=In%20somatic%20meditation%2C%20the%20focus

Watson, J. C. (2022, June). *Overview of pain*. MSD Manual Consumer Version. https://www.msdmanuals.com/home/brain

Waxenbaum, J. A., Reddy, V., & Varacallo, M. (2020, August 10). *Anatomy, autonomic nervous system*. National Library of Medicine; StatPearls Publishing. https://www.ncbi.nlm.nih.gov/books/NBK539845/#:~:text=The%20autonomic%20nervous%20system%20is

West, M. (n.d.). Vagus nerve QiGong exercises for emotional regulation [YouTube Video]. In *YouTube*. Retrieved September 28, 2022, from https://www.youtube.com/watch?v=ATHp6sa0418

Williams, E. (2021). This Posture Hack Instantly Deactivates The Stress Response. *Dragonfly Acupuncture & Massage*. https://acupuncturecarolina.com/blog/acupuncture-greenville-sc-this-posture-hack-instantly-deactivates-the-stress-response

Wim Hof Method. (n.d.). *Benefits of cold therapy*. Wim Hof Method. Retrieved September 26, 2022, from https://www.wimhofmethod.com/cold-therapy

WomensMedia. (2021, April 15). What the vagus nerve is and how to stimulate it for better mental health. *Forbes*. https://www.forbes.com/sites/womensmedia/2021/04/15/what-the-vagus-nerve-is-and-how-to-stimulate-it-for-better-mental-health/?sh=4e65ed926250

Yale Medicine. (2022). *Chronic stress*. Yale Medicine. https://www.yalemedicine.org/conditions/stress-

disorder#:~:text=%E2%80%A2A%20consistent%20se
nse%20of

Yuan, H., & Silberstein, S. D. (2015). Vagus nerve stimulation and headache. *Headache: The Journal of Head and Face Pain*, *57*, 29–33. https://doi.org/10.1111/head.12721

Printed in Great Britain
by Amazon